THE
Stash Plan

YOUR 21-DAY GUIDE TO SHED WEIGHT, FEEL GREAT, AND TAKE CHARGE OF YOUR HEALTH

Laura Prepon & Elizabeth Troy

TOUCHSTONE

NEW YORK   LONDON   TORONTO   SYDNEY   NEW DELHI

Touchstone
An Imprint of Simon & Schuster, Inc.
1230 Avenue of the Americas
New York, NY 10020

First Touchstone hardcover edition March 2016

For information about special discounts for bulk purchases, please contact Simon & Schuster Special
Sales at 1-866-506-1949 or business@simonandschuster.com.

The Simon & Schuster Speakers Bureau can bring authors to your live event.
For more information or to book an event, contact the Simon & Schuster Speakers Bureau at
1-866-248-3049 or visit our website at www.simonspeakers.com.

Interior design by Laura Palese

Photographs by Ray Kachatorian

Illustration (page 40) by Greg Miller

Illustrations (pages 43, 44, 47) by Thom Graves

Manufactured in the United States of America

5 7 9 10 8 6 4

Library of Congress Cataloging-in-Publication Data
Names: Prepon, Laura, 1980– author. | Troy, Elizabeth, (Integrative Nutritionist) author.
Title: The stash plan : your 21-day guide to shed weight, feel great, and take charge of your
health / Laura Prepon and Elizabeth Troy.
Description: New York : Touchstone, [2016] | Includes bibliographical references and index.
Identifiers: LCCN 2015034107|
Subjects: LCSH: Weight loss—Health aspects. | Nutrition. | Self-care, Health. | BISAC: HEALTH &
FITNESS / Healthy Living. | HEALTH & FITNESS / Weight Loss.
Classification: LCC RM222.2 .P69 2016 | DDC 613.2/5—dc23
LC record available at http://lccn.loc.gov/2015034107

ISBN 978-1-5011-2309-2
ISBN 978-1-5011-2314-6 (ebook)

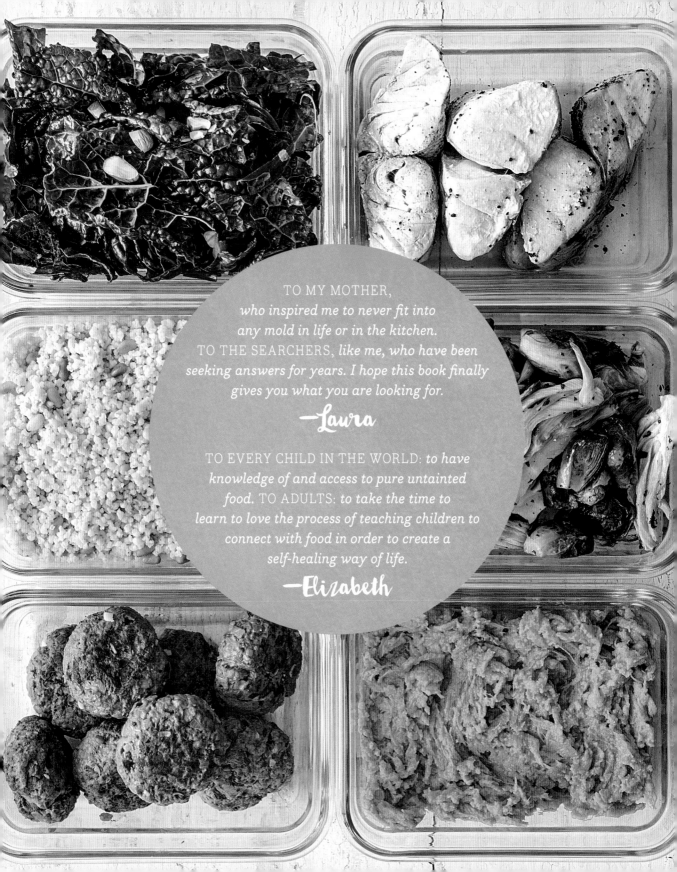

TO MY MOTHER,
*who inspired me to never fit into
any mold in life or in the kitchen.*
TO THE SEARCHERS, *like me, who have been
seeking answers for years. I hope this book finally
gives you what you are looking for.*

—*Laura*

TO EVERY CHILD IN THE WORLD: *to have
knowledge of and access to pure untainted
food.* TO ADULTS: *to take the time to
learn to love the process of teaching children to
connect with food in order to create a
self-healing way of life.*

—*Elizabeth*

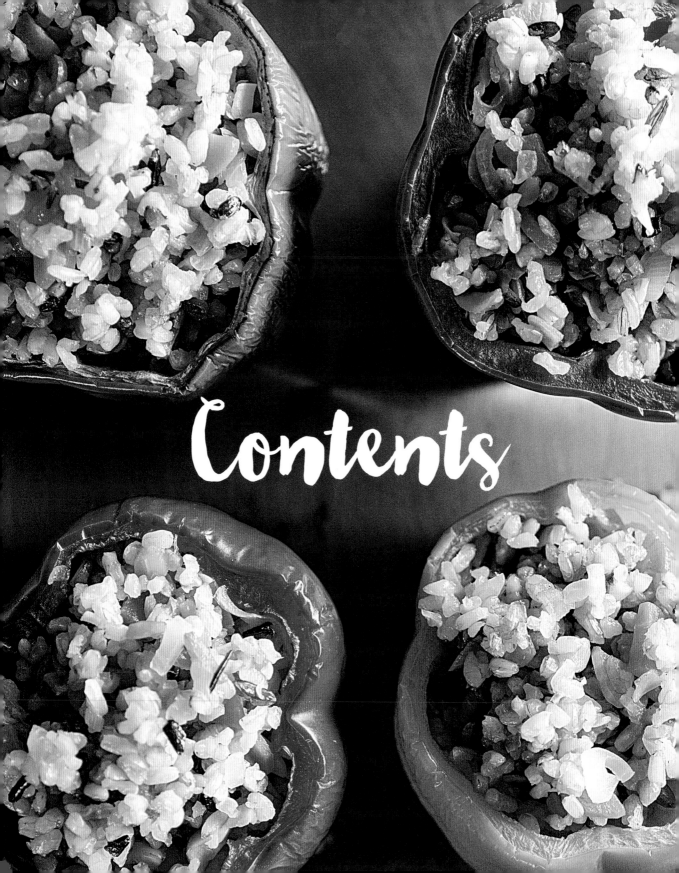

Contents

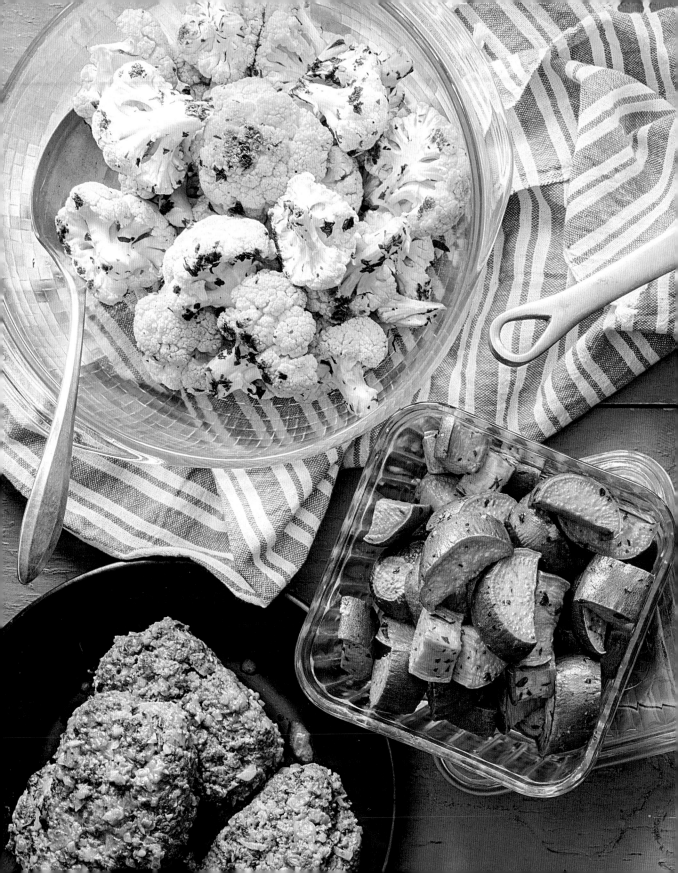

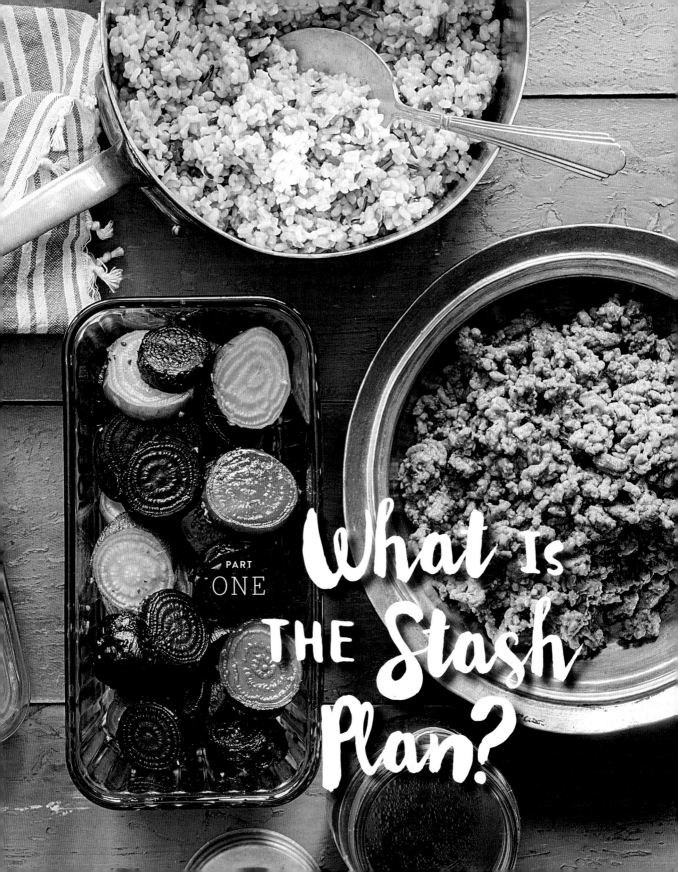

PART
ONE

What Is The Stash Plan?

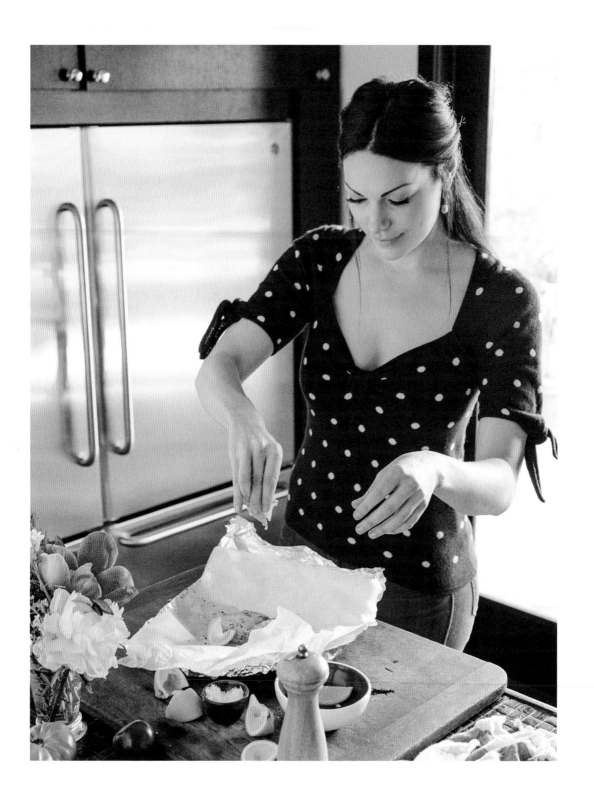

WHEN I RANG THE BUZZER

of a nondescript building in Manhattan's Chelsea neighborhood in July 2012, I had no idea that not only was I about to start a *journey* toward *wellness* that I desperately needed, but that this book would be the result! The buzzer belonged to Elizabeth Troy, an *integrative* nutritionist and well-being coach, and as we started the many months of the hard work of my *healing*, we talked endlessly about health and nutrition and Chinese Meridian Theory. These discussions have morphed into this part of the book. In *Chapter 1*, you'll learn our *stories* and what brought us together. In *Chapter 2*, we'll describe how the three pillars of the Stash Plan—the power of broth, making stashes that pack a nutritious punch, and *stretching* that opens the door to fat-burning—are so important. *Chapter 3* is a primer on the inner workings of your body, giving you information you might not have known before about the two key *organs* that make you a lean mean sexy machine—your gallbladder and your liver. You'll also learn how the modern diet and *environment* have created havoc on our bodies and what you can do to combat these problems. *Chapter 4* will teach you about the *best foods* to achieve the best you. *So let's get going!*

The STORY BEHIND THE Stash PLAN

chapter 1

•

Laura's Story

You might know me as Alex on Orange Is the
New Black, *or as Donna on* That '70s Show, *or
as Chelsea in* Are You There, Chelsea?
*But what most people don't know is that for years
I was at war with my body, and it affected every
aspect of my health and self-image . . . until
I finally figured out the solution.*

But first a bit about how I came to this place. Acting is my great love, and
I've been lucky enough to pursue my dream in the public eye for nearly
sixteen years. My other passion, one that far fewer know about, is cooking.
I grew up the youngest of five children, and my mother was a gourmet chef.
We always had friends over and even foreign exchange students staying in
our home. The principal of my school would joke with my mother, saying
that she was running a halfway house! The place where we would always
congregate was the kitchen, and I still love being in my own. I loved the
warm, comforting feeling of cooking for people and bonding over food, and
I've been hooked on cooking and entertaining ever since—so much so that
my friends teasingly call me Martha Stewart.

When I got to my early twenties, though, I started having issues with my digestion. I was gaining weight just when I really didn't need to be, and my energy levels started to plummet. Not to mention I was bloated and puffy most days. I had just started working on *That '70s Show* and was very worried, so I became obsessed with reading diet and health books, looking for answers. I have stacks of them in my house!

I'm the kind of person who likes to experience things for myself to make better-educated decisions, but this can be harmful when it comes to diets—because I would read these books and then *do* all the programs. This became problematic because these books, while well intentioned, often completely contradict one another. Sometimes the diets were so low-calorie I would fall off the wagon completely and eat something "bad" because I was so hungry. And despite my best efforts, after a week or so (if I even had enough energy and willpower to get that far), whatever plan I was trying would stop working. And then of course I would gain back more weight than before I even started.

This was the start of a cycle that was decidedly not healthy for me. I would be so upset at myself about the weight gain that I would pick up a different diet book and try *that* one. The same thing would happen: I would lose weight (usually water weight) for a few days; then my energy would plummet, then I would get so hungry I would ditch the plan and eat. It was a catch-22: It got to the point where I couldn't do my job or live a normal life, and I felt like I couldn't eat *anything* or I would gain weight.

I've done just about every diet there is, from Atkins and South Beach to cabbage soup cleanses. Food combining? Tried it. Caveman diet? Been there, done that. Alkaline diet? Bulletproof Coffee? Vegan? Atkins? Yup! I've done it all. Talk about contradictory advice! However, all of these efforts were futile.

And did I mention embarrassing, too? Once I was at a fancy power-lunch meeting at Bouchon (a very nice restaurant in Beverly Hills). I was sitting at the table with three producers, salivating as their amazingly delicious-looking plates of French food were delivered to the table. Meanwhile I was on a restrictive diet, so instead of ordering my own meal, I pulled a Tupperware container of cabbage soup out of my purse. It was a

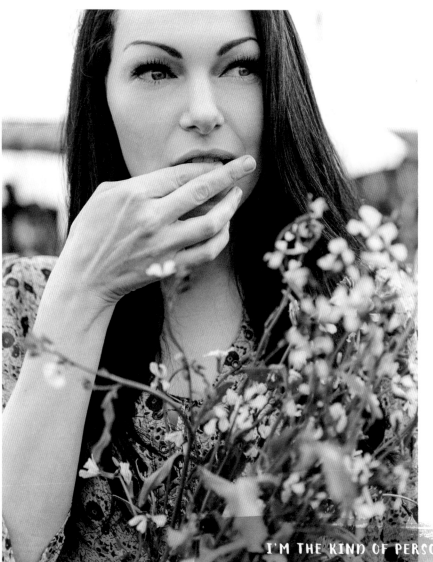

I'M THE KIND OF PERSON
WHO LIKES TO *experience*
THINGS FOR MYSELF.

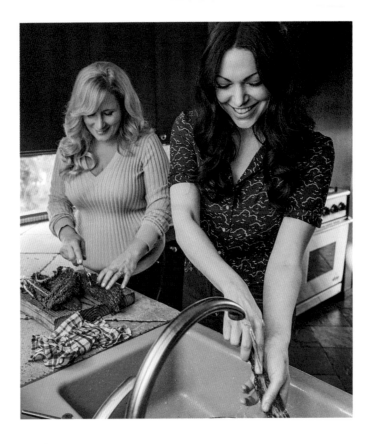

bit awkward to say the least, especially when the waiter bustled over to tell me I couldn't eat any food that wasn't prepared in their kitchen due to strict health codes. I was mortified . . . but I kept on trying.

During my next diet I was at a black-tie event at the Beverly Hilton. I was so hungry I snuck into the bathroom, the train of my gorgeous gown flowing behind me, and hid in a stall like a teenager sneaking a cigarette in between classes. But I wasn't grabbing a smoke; I was trying to quickly scarf down some diet-approved food out of sight of any waiters or guests. I wasn't going to risk the health-code warning again, but I was so hungry I knew that if I didn't eat *something* I was going to chew on Lady Gaga's hat. On this particular diet I was instructed to eat only six crackers per day, along with small amounts of carefully weighed food. Luckily for me, my clutch was just big enough to hold my iPhone, a lip-gloss tube, and the tiny bit of food I was allowed to chew on for "dinner."

The last diet I tried before finding my nutritionist, Elizabeth Troy, really did a number on me. A doctor I consulted prescribed injections of HCG (a hormone secreted by pregnant women) to trick my body into thinking it was pregnant. The idea was that these injections (which I did myself every morning) would cause my body to burn stored body fat to support the "baby." This regimen was accompanied by a starvation-level 500-calorie-per-day diet. I know what you're thinking, and yes, it's just as crazy as it sounds, but I was willing to try anything. When I stopped it, not only did I gain all the weight back, but my hormones were completely out of whack.

I KNEW I NEEDED *expert* ADVICE.

As a working actress, I was partial to crash diets because my schedule was always in flux and jobs can come up suddenly. I'd get a call about a photo shoot scheduled for two days hence, or a job that would start shooting in a mere three days. When I got the awesome news that I'd been cast in *Orange Is the New Black*, I had only fourteen hours' notice to move from Los Angeles to New York City and start filming a day and a half later—and my first scene was a shower scene! I was so nervous about my figure, I think I starved myself for a full forty hours. My poor body was so confused it didn't know what I was going to do to it next.

Because I was so unsure about what to do to get my body to feel good and look the way I wanted, I knew I needed expert advice. Over the years, I went from doctor to doctor in search of answers. One told me I had Hashimoto's thyroiditis, an autoimmune condition of the thyroid. The next told me that I didn't have Hashimoto's, but that my thyroid was still out of whack and I needed pills—for life. Another told me my adrenal glands were "blown out" from stress, and that's why I couldn't burn fat, yet the next told me I wasn't burning fat because my hormone levels were that of a postmenopausal woman. One told me I had leaky gut. One charged me thousands of dollars for food-allergy testing, and then gave me forty different supplements to take. Another thought I had mono.

I also went to nutritionists who were very good at listening to me and believing that there was something wrong, but their plans often became

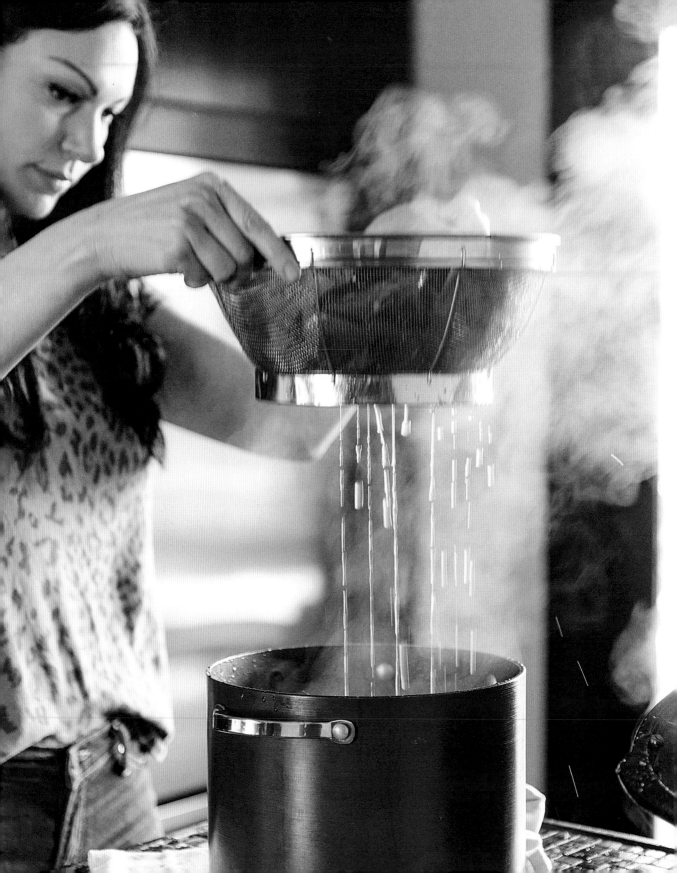

contradictory and confusing as well. One took my temperature and joked that I had the "temperature of a dead person." (I may be pale with long black hair and look like Elvira, but I certainly didn't want the core body temperature of a vampire!) He explained that low body temperature equals low metabolism, and had me eat a ton of carbs to get it to go up—but the only thing that moved up was the dial on the scale. I even went to a shaman-type nutritionist who shook maracas over my head as she cast some kind of spell. As you could imagine, that didn't work either.

At the same time as my consulting these experts, I was working out like a maniac. I'm the opposite of lazy—I always worked out more than anyone I knew. I used to do triple workout sessions in one day; first a kickboxing class, then a run, and then I'd lift weights at night. My muscles were toned, but I wasn't strong (and certainly not as strong as I should have been with all that exercising). And I never felt energized or vibrant after my workouts. And one thing was really weird—I never got sore, even though I spent hours taxing my muscles. My body was so numb that it was literally giving up on me.

Every day became a struggle. I could barely get up for my early calls. I was increasingly lethargic and struggling to lose weight. This was a huge problem because in my business there is this crazy pressure, as you know, to look a certain way—but rain or shine, no matter how I felt, I still had to go to work and sometimes shoot for up to seventeen hours a day. I would drink so much coffee (sometimes an entire pot before noon) to keep me standing that my stomach felt as if there were a hole being burned in it from all the churning acid. Here I was, with the most amazing job I have ever dreamed of, and I was having an extremely hard time just getting through the day.

Can you believe that all of this took place over a span of *fifteen* years? I invested an incredible amount of time (and an insane amount of money), but no matter what I tried, I felt like I was trapped in a daily battle with my body. The fight left me exhausted, self-conscious, and unable to enjoy the good that life was sending my way. Nothing seemed to help, because nobody could figure out what, specifically, was wrong with me.

And then a miracle happened. A friend told me about this healer named Elizabeth Troy. I asked what specifically she does, and my friend just said, "it's kind of hard to explain, but you've never done anything like it." Intrigued and never one to shy away from a new diet, regimen, or expert, I reached out right away—only to hear that she was so popular she wasn't taking on any new clients. But after some persistent follow-up on my end , Elizabeth said she'd see me right away. I had an intuitive feeling that I had to get to her as quickly as possible, and I started counting down the days till our first session in July 2012.

When I arrived at her studio in Chelsea in New York City, Elizabeth greeted me warmly. She had such a calm, maternal, and compassionate aura about her, but she was this badass New Yorker at the same time. We instantly bonded. I then proceeded to have my mind blown with the information I was about to learn.

Elizabeth began by explaining that conventional medical practices don't understand precisely how modern life and diet are adversely affecting the gallbladder and liver—the two most important organs for the regulation of energy in your body.

"What do you mean?" I asked. I had learned in school what most people learn about the human body: mostly the central nervous system and the circulatory system. I felt I had a good understanding of the human body, especially because I had educated myself so much on the subject, but had no idea how vital the functioning of the gallbladder and liver were not only for producing energy and burning fat but for actually nourishing the body.

"I'll explain as I get to work," she said, gesturing to several large mats on the floor of her studio. She then told me that I should lie down on one. As I lay on my stomach, she started walking on my legs and back—which I already knew was an essential component of Thai massage—in order to get a feel for my body and figure out what was going on.

Have you ever gone for a massage or facial and realized the minute you felt the therapist's hands on you that they were the hands of a healer? That's how I felt when Elizabeth started walking on my calves and the back of my thighs and told me about Chinese Meridian Theory. I didn't know much about it, but Elizabeth explained that she'd tweaked its fundamental precepts to create her own program, called the Muscle Meridian Method, for her clients. She explained that all energy starts in the gallbladder and

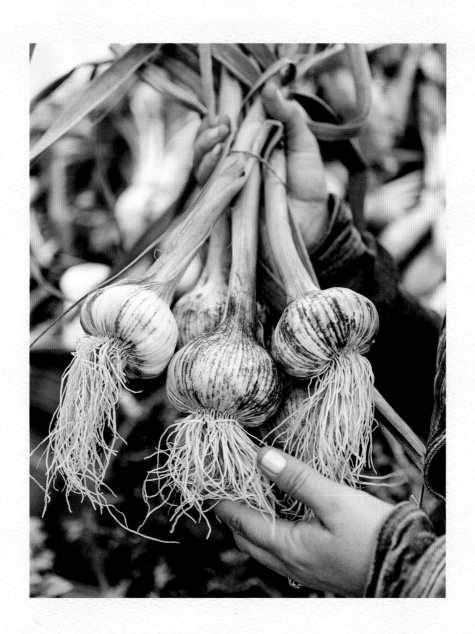

liver, and that it is crucial to get these two organs to function properly before dealing with any other health issues.

"In traditional Chinese medicine, it is believed that qi, or your energy, 'originates' in the gallbladder and liver. This is true for nearly every species," she told me as her feet gently pressed on my muscles. It didn't hurt at all; in fact, it was very soothing.

"The gallbladder and liver work together synergistically, and when they're functioning normally, then *all* the internal organs are primed to work effectively. But when the gallbladder and liver are blocked, all of the other organs will be blocked, too, leading to a cascade effect of problematic weight and health issues."

I then learned that due to the perils of modern food—particularly GMOs, or genetically modified foods—and the stresses of modern life, our gallbladders and livers can be taxed beyond belief. When these two organs can't function properly, we become overweight, bloated, and mentally foggy—about as energetic as a worn-out battery. No wonder I was drinking an entire pot of coffee every day.

I had always prepped my food and cooked in bulk so I could bring my meals to work. Because my digestion was so sensitive, I never knew how my body was going to react to food. Elizabeth explained that if your gallbladder and liver are stuck, these super-stressed-out organs are no longer able to metabolize food properly, even if you're eating good, nutritious food. This is particularly true for fats; without a healthy gallbladder and liver, your body has a lot of trouble converting the fat (even healthy fats) in your diet into energy, so all the fat in my diet was instead getting stored in places where it shouldn't be stored. As time went on, I'd get more and more inflamed. My body just wasn't capable of absorbing the nutrients from all that healthy food I was eating.

This was a eureka moment for me. I finally understood why I was always hungry and always feeling puffy and unwell, even

THIS WAS A *eureka* MOMENT FOR ME. I FINALLY *understood* WHY I WAS ALWAYS HUNGRY AND *always* FEELING PUFFY AND UNWELL.

though I was eating "nutritious" food. My body was literally starved, because it wasn't able to properly absorb the nutrients I desperately needed, so it was constantly holding on to fat for survival.

She also told me that the gallbladder and liver are the first two organs to be taxed by toxins, thanks to high-fat, high-sugar processed foods; environmental pollutants; bad farming practices; overuse of prescriptive medications; poor storage and transport of foods; unhealthy cooking practices; and the stress we all deal with on a daily basis.

By this point, Elizabeth was walking up and down my spine and very gently probing around my shoulder blades with her feet. She said, "It's impossible to burn fat efficiently and create a lean, *Avatar*-like body if the gallbladder and the liver can't do their jobs."

"I can't believe it," I said. Nobody had ever explained this to me before. "It's like the key piece of information about my health—and the health of who knows how many others struggling with the same things—has been missing."

I went on to describe my crazy exercise regime, and Elizabeth shook her head, telling me that kind of pounding I'd been giving myself was precisely the *worst* thing I could do. What I needed to do instead, she said, was to focus on stretching exercises to keep the energy flowing properly in my body, and certain kinds of aerobic exercises (rebounding on a mini trampoline and running were okay, but the StairMaster and squats were no-no's) to help my lymphatic system flush out toxins and reduce the bloat. I couldn't believe that all those hours spent every day trying to make myself fit might actually have been hurting me!

At that point, Elizabeth had me sit up and we kept on talking. She explained how her stretching works, and how the first step in the eating plan she was going to devise for me was to drink nutritious broths several times a day. "The micronutrients in these broths will assimilate into your body right away and heal you at a cellular level," she told me. "We need to get your body absorbing nutrients, first and foremost."

I'd been to many practitioners over the years, but this was the first time I'd ever heard anything new and *different*. That this was a plan that might actually work.

WITHIN ONLY
a few days,
THERE WAS AN
astonishing
EFFECT ON MY
energy

After that first session, I practically ran to the butcher to buy the organic bones Elizabeth told me to get, and I made an enormous pot of delicious beef broth that night. Within only a few days, there was an astonishing effect on my energy.

Elizabeth and I continued to work together as my body and health were transformed. My body was in such a weakened state when I came to her that I had a lot of work ahead of me, but I was willing to do all of it. It didn't hurt that Elizabeth was so supportive and impressed with my tenacity. She taught me exactly what to eat, when to eat it, and why so I could get my gallbladder and liver to function properly. No diet book had ever explained that when these two organs aren't working correctly, you can't possibly burn fat and keep weight off. Like so many others, I had a low-functioning gallbladder and a "stuck" liver.

Until what became the Stash Plan got them unstuck!

Two years into our work together, I was feeling great for what seemed like the first time in my adult life. My energy was up. I felt toned and strong. I fit into my wardrobe without all the angst and deprivation I'd become used to. My skin looked so good that one tabloid doctor insisted I'd had a facelift. Nope, it was just the effects of the collagen in the bone broth and the healing that was happening in my body, from the inside out.

And because the one thing that hadn't changed in my life was my busy schedule, Elizabeth and I had figured out a way to make this way of eating not just tasty but also convenient. We were both batch-cooking pros, so cooking in bulk evolved as the crux of the Stash Plan. I'd do one big cooking session, twice a week. My bone broth could simmer on the stovetop or even in a slow cooker during the day or overnight. I could take the healthy, simple meals with me on the go—my "stash" of good food could come with me everywhere. And if I found myself at a fancy restaurant, I had the tools and knowledge to make healthy choices out in the real world, too.

One day Elizabeth and I had another one of those eureka moments. I had always wanted to write a book, one about food that was inspired

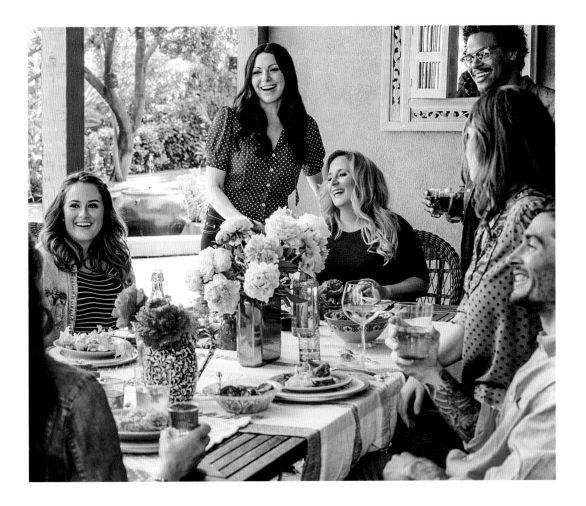

by my mother and her love of cooking. And I'd been thinking a lot about the specific foods I was eating and how they made me feel. "If the Muscle Meridian Method had such a profound effect on my life, couldn't we help so many more people if we could take this message wider?" I asked her.

We looked at each other in excitement. From there, we fine-tuned our work together and created the Stash Plan—our targeted eating and stretching plan that is as convenient and fun as it is life-changing. The Stash Plan is going to do for you what it did for me. Read on, and Elizabeth and I will show you how.

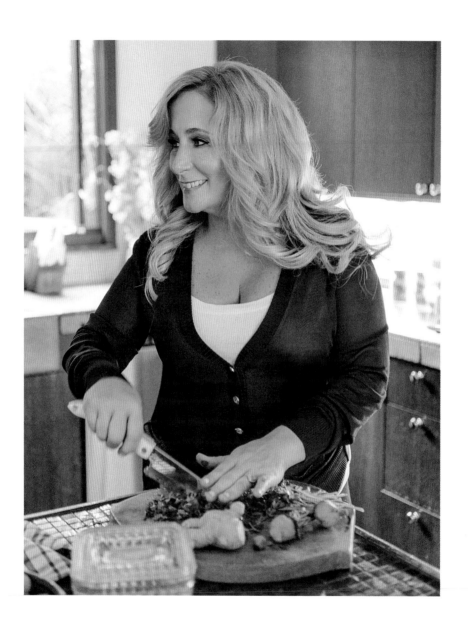

Elizabeth's Story

I decided to become an educator and a healer after a terrible car accident in my twenties derailed my burgeoning law school career—and almost took my life. As I recovered, I gained a new appreciation for not only traditional Western medicine but also complementary Eastern medicine—both of which combined to heal me and put me on the path I continue on today.

I received my master's degree in teaching from Teachers College at Columbia University and became a certified teacher of yoga and Thai muscle massage. I'm also a registered practitioner of functional medicine and nutrition with Metagenics, a certified nutritionist with the Institute for Integrative Nutrition, and a practitioner of Chinese Meridian Theory. I consider it a great honor that Columbia University has me on their list of top complementary medicine practitioners in the country.

Today I'm based in New York City and work with an amazing and impressive array of people, including Laura. But my practice started out *much* more modestly! In 1997, I opened a little studio on Main Street in Fishkill, New York, a small town in a conservative area that was home to the largest IBM plant in the world. My studio was a room that could comfortably fit six people on stretching mats on the floor. I literally wrote my phone number, 896-YOGA, on blank pieces of paper because no one would have had a clue what stretching for your gallbladder and liver meant! Shortly after I opened the doors, my daughter was feeling sick one morning and I was late getting to the studio. As I approached the studio, I saw a line of people and thought there was a parade going on. I quickly realized they were waiting to get into my nine a.m. class! That day I walked down the street to get a bigger space.

LIKE MY clients, I WORK AT BECOMING healthier EVERY DAY.

Within two weeks I had over fifty clients, and within a month that grew to a hundred and fifty. I didn't want to leave the great location on or near Main Street and was fortunate to have found a space on the next block, but I was concerned about how big it was—over 2,000 square feet. I took a deep breath and went for it, and within two months I had three hundred clients, eighteen classes running, and was doing upward of twenty-five private sessions a week. I had no advertising—it was all word of mouth.

I started each week teaching about the gallbladder and liver, and I researched which foods were the most beneficial for their optimal functioning, which weren't, and how they could best be prepared. As my practice grew, with more clients wanting to deal with their weight issues, I spent even more time on nutrition. I knew all the health issues and weight issues I was seeing were connected—but this was in 1998, when few people were discussing digestion, let alone gut health or GMOs, or how to eat properly for the health of your internal organs—and I knew I had to think outside the box. By 1999, I was in an even larger studio and started holding workshops and trainings in New York City, the Hamptons, Boston, Washington, DC, California, and Topsail Island, North Carolina.

As my practice continued to expand over the years, I was able to successfully treat thousands of patients with autoimmune disorders, weight problems, fertility issues, skin disorders such as eczema and allergies, and other emotional and physical ailments. All of my clients are unique, from world-class professional and Olympic athletes to titans of Wall Street to dancers, artists, salesmen, other working professionals, teenagers with

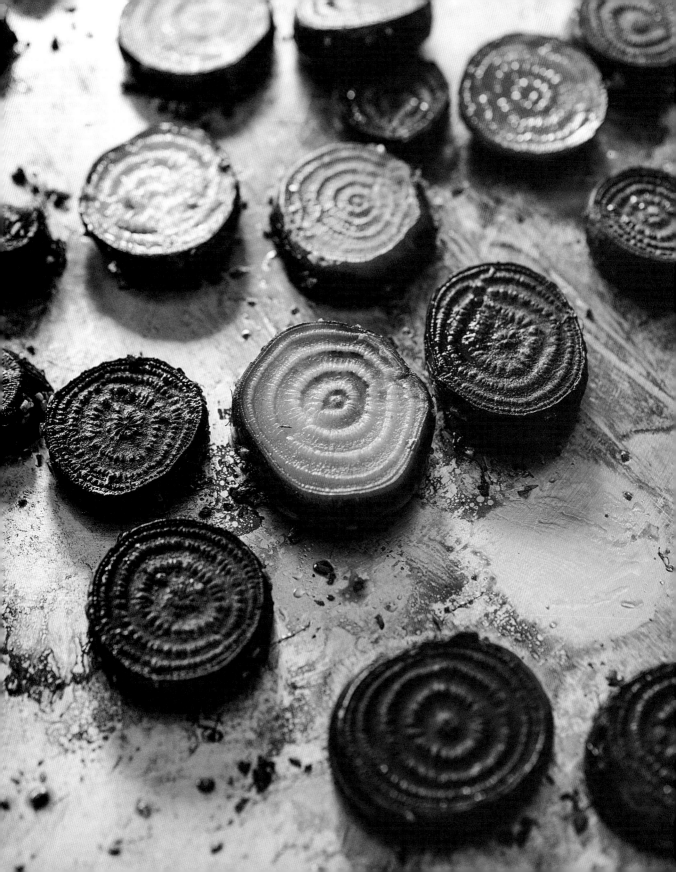

terrible skin and weight problems, and moms (and dads) and their children with learning and emotional issues.

I also began to notice a terrifying rise of autoimmune diseases, not just in the general population and with my clients but in my own life. Then in 2007 I was diagnosed with Lyme disease. Actually, I'd been misdiagnosed, and by the time I went to an internist who could test me with more accuracy, I was very sick, with extreme exhaustion, numbness in my limbs, confusion and short-term memory loss, and a compromised immune system.

Lyme disease attacks the liver first, by burying its spirochetes (bacteria) into the deepest part of the liver. I could feel the disease wreaking havoc on my liver—and through it, my whole body. I needed three months of oral antibiotics followed by six months of intravenous antibiotics to start to heal. The intravenous antibiotics came in an eight-ounce bag that hung off my hip with a catheter going into a primary main vein, and I started wearing oversize layered shirts to conceal it. All my clients were coming to me for healing, yet here I was, needing this healing more than they did. That's when I knew I had to figure this out in a scientific way. My clients and family were relying on me, and something had to change.

I knew about the muscles and the exterior body, but this bout of Lyme disease opened my eyes to seeing things from the inside out versus from the outside in. It brought it full circle for me. I found that the healthier I could keep my gallbladder and liver, the more I could manage the disease. Eventually, I was able to take myself off every medication and rebuild my ravaged immune system with what we now call the Stash Plan.

Like my clients, I work at becoming healthier every day. All of us have seen how food and drink can have amazingly positive effects on gallbladders and livers, clearing and energizing the body so that the spirit can flourish. My clients all lost weight. They all saw their immune systems strengthen, their energy levels soar, and their mental and spiritual health improve. They all found a better balance in their lives, bodies, career, family, and community.

I also noticed that progressive hospitals were paying more attention to complementary care with traditional medicine. The Hospital for Special Surgery in New York and Connecticut is now putting patients on

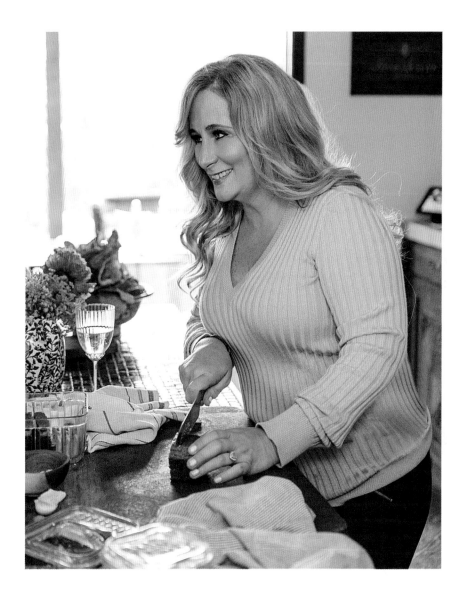

anti-inflammatory diets for two weeks prior to and after surgery, for example, diets similar in concept to the Stash Plan's broths.

So I looked into a fellowship program at the Center Institute for Research and Education in Integrative Medicine through the Department of Integrative Medicine at Mount Sinai Beth Israel Hospital. I was welcomed into the program at the end of 2014—they were intrigued by my diverse background in nutrition and hands-on healing—and currently work along-side medical doctors, psychiatrists, acupuncturists, and family therapists.

Functional medicine is about taking the patient as a whole. Its practitioners know now that traditional medicine is not the only answer to these new diseases. You need to heal different aspects of the person in order for him or her to get well. The other medical professionals in my group were so supportive of my work and information, in fact, that they actually started canceling sessions when I wasn't able to be there, because I was traveling to and from Los Angeles to work with Laura and other clients. We soon set up a system so that when we did our case studies (complicated patient cases, part of every practitioner's workload), I could give my protocol for the patients when I was not in New York. It is heartening not only to be a part of this fellowship but also to see the medical community becoming more open-minded to complementary ways of helping to heal their patients.

To date, I have treated over three thousand clients and trained over three hundred healers in the Muscle Meridian Method. I've had many clients with tough health issues—eating disorders, irritable bowel syndrome, multiple sclerosis, ADD/ADHD, autism, arthritis, and allergies—but I had never had one like Laura before. One hot July day, in walked this powerful woman with great beauty and a vibrant, powerful personality, and yet, as I soon discovered, she had absolutely no strength in her body.

The first thing I do with my private clients, as with Laura, is walk on them, to feel their tissues. This allows me to ascertain if there is a lot of fluid, or if their tendons are too tight, among other things. While I'm walking, I ask everyone how it feels. Some people are so inflamed that they literally can't bear any of my weight and I have to hop off. One client, a six-foot-two man who weighed 220 pounds, was so sensitive to the touch that when I was standing on him, near his shoulders, as I did my Thai massage techniques, he literally tried to bite my toe.

Not Laura. She lay on the mat, relaxed and at ease, and didn't feel a thing. Not one little footstep. She was *totally* numb. I felt like if I wasn't paying heed, I could put my feet right through her.

As I felt my way up her spine, I became increasingly alarmed, because Laura had described the intensity of her daily workouts to me, so I expected to find a body that was taut with strong muscles. Instead, her intense weight training and cardio had left hard knots under her bones. She was *so* stuck in *so* many areas of her body that it had become impossible for any energy to flow through properly.

I quickly started telling Laura about fascia, the connective tissue in your body. Her knotted fascia was tougher and more gnarled than that of practically any other client I'd ever worked with. I explained that gnarled-up fascia stops qi from moving, and that my targeted stretching would help unkink it, along with the food plan I'd be giving her.

I quietly kept talking, as something very serious was going on. Laura ate so well and worked out so much that the slackness of her muscles combined with the knots just shouldn't have been there. I quickly realized I had to focus on her lower body to get her gallbladder and liver meridians to start firing. Otherwise, she would become even more ill than she was already.

It took only a few days of specific eating, broths, and targeted stretching for Laura to respond. Soon, as she started to heal, her energy skyrocketed. In addition, I made her stop her daily weight training and kickboxing and get on a mini trampoline and rebound instead, as that would get her lymphatic system moving. Within only a few weeks, this amazing woman who'd been perilously close to complete collapse was finally on the road to wellness.

What Laura learned was this: When you eat what your gallbladder and liver need, this fires your meridians and unblocks energy . . . which in turn stimulates the organ's function . . . which causes a cascade of amazing effects on your body and mind. It's a plan that really works, and once you learn how to then cook healthy foods yourself and take your "stash" on the road with you, eating well becomes not a fad, but a lifestyle.

Once the Stash Plan way of eating and stretching becomes a regular part of your life, your energy will continue to soar as Laura's did. You'll finally be able to metabolize foods for maximum nutrition. Your body will shift and improve, and you'll begin to notice many other positive changes in your life. Noticing these boosts in your confidence and clearheadedness will be one of the most exciting rewards for your commitment to Stashing.

·

Our Mission

Now that you know how we came together, you have a better understanding of our mission. Elizabeth always says, "If you educate, people will motivate."

We want to educate the world so that no one would ever have to endure what we have endured in order to figure it out—and so that people everywhere can finally heal. The kind of yo-yo dieting made so popular by the latest new diet trend, and the types of botched treatments Laura was told to do for years, need to stop. It's insanity. This book will help you to make clear, informed choices about your eating, your body, and the good health you deserve to have.

We've been working for years to create this book—to make it as user-friendly as possible, to make these concepts easy to understand, and to finally give you answers. We can't imagine our lives without our Stashes! And hopefully, soon you won't either.

You deserve to eat food that hasn't been tainted with chemicals or genetically modified without any testing. You deserve to know exactly what's on your plate. You deserve to have your nagging symptoms, lack of energy, emotional numbness, and extra pounds gone and out of your life for good!

SO, LET'S GET STASHING!

·

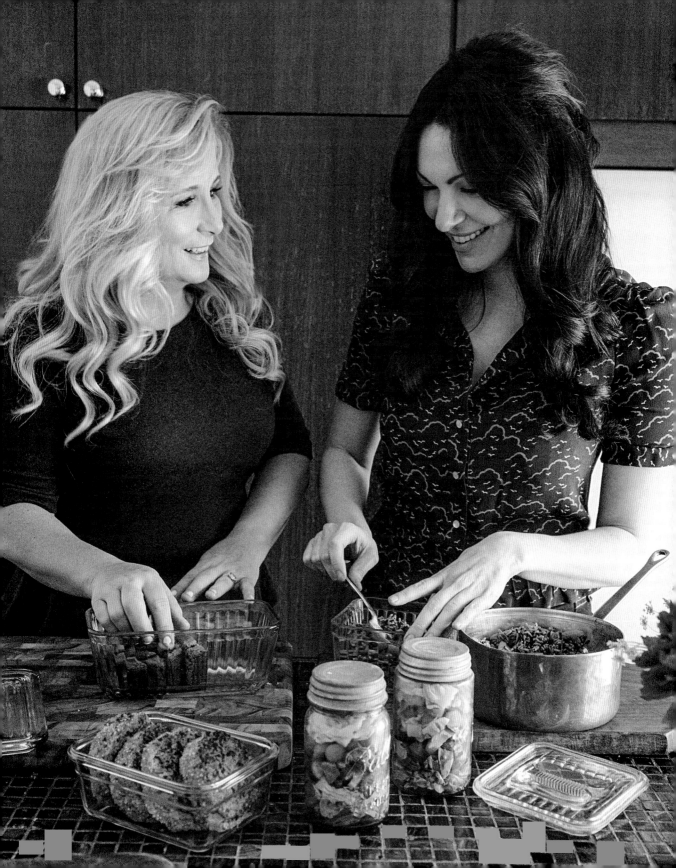

How the
STASH PLAN
WORKS

chapter 2

How does the Stash Plan work? By unblocking your stuck gallbladder and liver in a unique way, through food and movement, and then by giving you the tools to cook and eat that food anywhere, anytime, for maximum health and healing.

Unblocked energy creates harmony in the body, so your body will naturally detox and heal itself. As you become more attuned to your body's food needs:

- **You will gain energy and lose weight naturally,** without struggles or restrictive dieting. This will happen as soon as you start eating non-GMO, organic, and grass-fed food and hydrating yourself properly in the targeted steps you'll soon read about.

  The processed/packaged foods that are unfortunately staples of the average American diet are virtually anything that comes in a box, bag, jar, or can—essentially food that has been tampered with by canning, cooking, freezing, dehydrating, or milling. These foods promote weight gain and chronic disease because they are high in sugar, fructose, refined carbohydrates, and artificial ingredients (which your body perceives as foreign substances), and low in live nutrients and fiber. They also trigger insulin resistance and chronic inflammation, hallmarks of most chronic and/or serious diseases.

  Processed and packaged foods are designed by their manufacturers to make you overeat; they also encourage food cravings, leading to weight gain. But when you eat fresh, wholesome food, your body will no longer need to figure out where to put any foreign substances (usually stuffed away in your body's fat to protect your organs from danger). As a result, you will naturally lose those unwanted pounds—and keep them off.

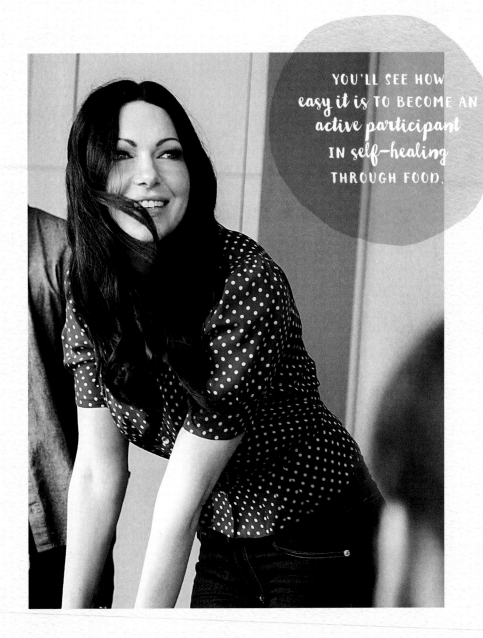

YOU'LL SEE HOW *easy it is* TO BECOME AN *active participant* IN *self-healing* THROUGH FOOD.

- You will notice a big decrease in appetite. You'll literally eat less food on the Stash Plan—not because we restrict you, but because you won't want to gorge yourself. The cravings for junk food will disappear and you'll save money not buying expensive and unhealthy packaged foods.

  We'll teach you exactly what to eat and drink and what to avoid. For example, avocados help the gallbladder metabolize and burn fat; beets help create new blood, so the liver can filter out the old blood faster and more easily. You'll see how easy it is to become an active participant in self-healing through food.

- You won't want to cheat! As you become accustomed to your Stashes, you probably won't want to eat anything else—but when you do, go ahead and enjoy it. If you aim for a realistic 80 percent Stash/20 percent your-favorite-everything-else, you are still going to reap all the benefits and have no inclination to "cheat" as you would on so many other diets. The Stash Plan is cheat-proof!

- You will prevent illness by rebuilding your immune system. Your Stash meals (including the delicious bone broth you'll learn how to make—it's easy!) will rebuild you from the inside out. Not only will you feel better but your skin will glow with vitality.

- You will rid yourself of inflammation and even see that pesky cellulite disappear. Once you start healing your insides, you'll be amazed at the transformation of your outside, in terms of both pounds on the scale and inches around the waist, hips, arms, and elsewhere.

- You will learn the right way to exercise, stretch, and breathe so that you get fitter faster—and never waste time in the gym again. This is active resistance stretching designed to open up your energy pathways and keep your joints functioning correctly.

- You'll improve your state of mind. The Stash Plan helps you to pull neurotoxins from the central nervous system and gets the cerebral spinal fluid unstuck from the sacrum, the area of your lower back between your hipbones. This gives you mental clarity and can even alleviate depression.

SO WHAT IS
the Stash Plan?

THERE ARE THREE synergistically charged elements in the Stash Plan: Stashes, broths, and targeted stretching.

1. A Stash is, literally, your treasure trove of eating. Twice a week you will cook foods in bulk, and these foods will be the basis of your meal building for the next three days. Each week's Stash is a macro- and micronutrient balanced meal that includes snacks—meaning no deprivation. Not only are these foods specifically geared toward unblocking your liver and gallbladder, but cooking your own food is an important part of the program. We will show you exactly how to build all your meals from your Stash so you always have fun new combinations. They are unbelievably delicious and easy to prepare, even if you think you don't know how to boil water!

   Each week you will have two Stash-up days. On Stash-up Day One (Sunday), you will make foods for Monday through Wednesday; on Stash-up Day Two (Wednesday) you will make your Stash for Thursday through Saturday. Sunday will be your day off from Stashes, as long as you eat all-organic, non-GMO food and have your broth.

   You will build three nutritious and delicious meals and two snacks from your prepared Stash each morning. Each Stash contains two proteins, two carbohydrates, and two veggies. You will also have what we call "hand grabbers," items that you can grab to add to your meals as well as use to make snacks. Examples of hand grabbers are avocados, nuts, and berries. It will take less than ten minutes to create your meals. You will also be astonished at how much free time you'll have when you Stash, and your food bills will go down dramatically, too.

2. Broth is quite simply the nutritional fountain of youth! It's the main reason people will ask you why you look so much younger and more vibrant once you start the Stash Plan. Each Stash is accompanied by a broth (beef, chicken, fish, or a vegetable option if you prefer), the ideal

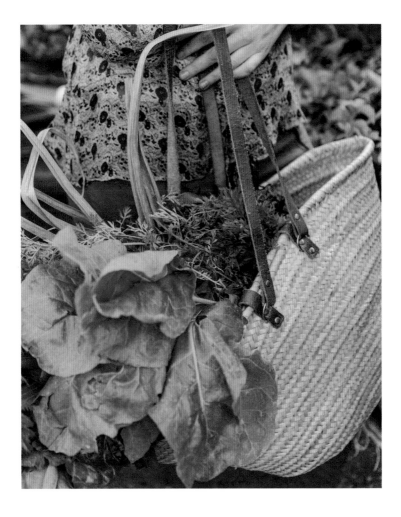

food to rejuvenate and detoxify your body. Broths are collagen rich and full of micronutrients from beef bones, whole chickens, whole fish, and vegetables. As micronutrients can't be stored in your body, you need to consume them every day. They include minerals such as iron, cobalt, copper, and zinc; enzymes; and vitamins A, Bs, C, and D. Broths are incredibly simple to make and powerhouses of healing nutrition as they repair your body at the microlevel. They unstick the liver and gallbladder by helping them to filter chemicals, preservatives, bacteria, and viruses from blood.

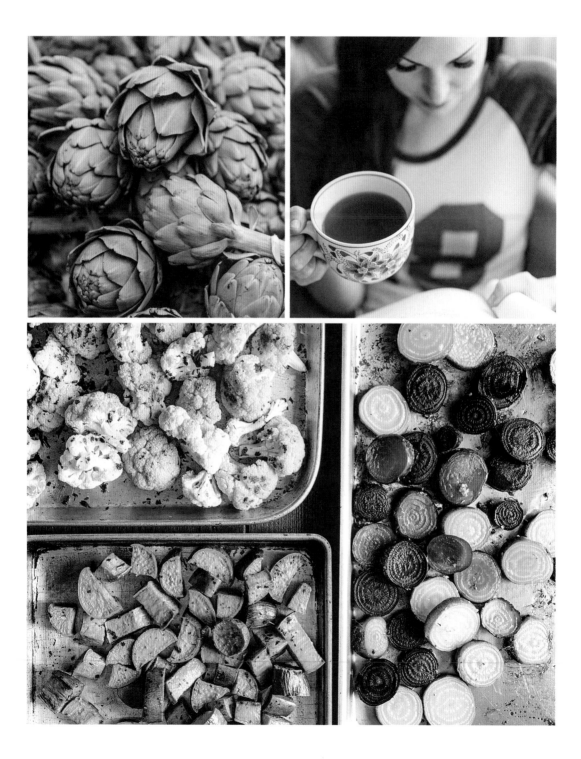

Your broths are part of these snacks and/or meals—think of them as your daily vitamin and pick-me-up in a cup that accompanies the program.

3. The stretching you'll be doing will ignite your meridians, bringing more energy to your gallbladder and liver and making them function better. This means you can finally burn fat like you're supposed to! These stretches take only twenty minutes a day, supercharging your qi. You will feel calm, energized, and toned, and you will feel inspired—knowing that you are going to be burning fat for hours to come.

These aren't the typical ways you'd stretch before or after a workout. They are specific movements that target these energy pathways and unblock your fascia, an incredibly important part of your body, one overlooked by most health professionals until recently. Fascia is the connective tissue in your body, that protective sheath that holds your muscles in place. When you don't work out or stretch correctly, and when you eat processed foods, packaged foods, or nonorganic foods containing a slew of chemicals, fascia gets gnarled up and stops qi from moving. If you've ever gotten a massage and a knot that gets pushed around makes you flinch, that's "stuck" fascia. Toxins get stuck in these fascia clusters (notably, causing cellulite as well).

These unique stretches lengthen and contract your muscles while you resist. The result helps break up these clusters and get the qi moving properly, allowing your liver and gallbladder to burn fat and flush out toxins as they were meant to.

The Stash Stretches ignite the meridians to your gallbladder and liver for maximum fat-burning and digestion and take only minutes a day to do so.

Sounds simple, right? Because it is!

The Stash Plan will literally heal you from the inside out. Even better, it takes only twenty-one days!

> The Stash Stretches IGNITE THE meridians TO YOUR GALLBLADDER AND LIVER FOR maximum FAT-BURNING AND digestion.

Our plan isn't just doable—it's *fun*. We are firm believers in *fun* in all aspects of life, especially with food. We won't say, "Never eat this!" or "Never drink that!" Aim for an 80/20 balance, where 80 percent is optimized for your body and 20 percent is whatever else you want to eat. If you're craving a doughnut, eat it and enjoy it. If you're going out to dinner, order what you want and have a drink or two if you're so inclined; enjoy every drop. Stressing yourself about eating causes more stress in your body and makes you toxic!

Eating the right food truly *can* transform your life.

True healing isn't just about physical health. It's about every aspect of being human. We want to help everyone find their way, successfully empowered to develop their own self-created healing through the Stash Plan.

We believe there are five things you can never have enough of: health, love, friendship, knowledge, and self-esteem. We consider self-esteem the engine, and the self-created healing of the Stash Plan the fuel for that engine. You'll soon discover that as you use the Stash Plan, all five things you cannot have enough of keep growing and growing! You'll also find that the Stashes will simplify and improve your eating so much that you won't be able to imagine life without them.

You deserve to eat food that hasn't been tainted with chemicals or genetically modified without any testing. You deserve to know exactly what's on your plate. You deserve to have your nagging symptoms, lack of energy, emotional numbness, and extra pounds gone and out of your life for good! You deserve to look and feel your best.

We can't wait to teach you how easy it is to Stash. As soon as you start, you'll be on the path toward a lifetime of better eating, vibrant energy, and the body you know you deserve. So go ahead and dump all those diet books on the recycling pile, toss the ineffective supplements, and cancel the expensive appointments with dubious medical practitioners. You won't need them anymore. The Stash Plan is a revolutionary new system that targets and ignites your gallbladder and liver, the gatekeepers to your best self. It's like no other plan in the world.

Are you ready? Let's get Stashing!

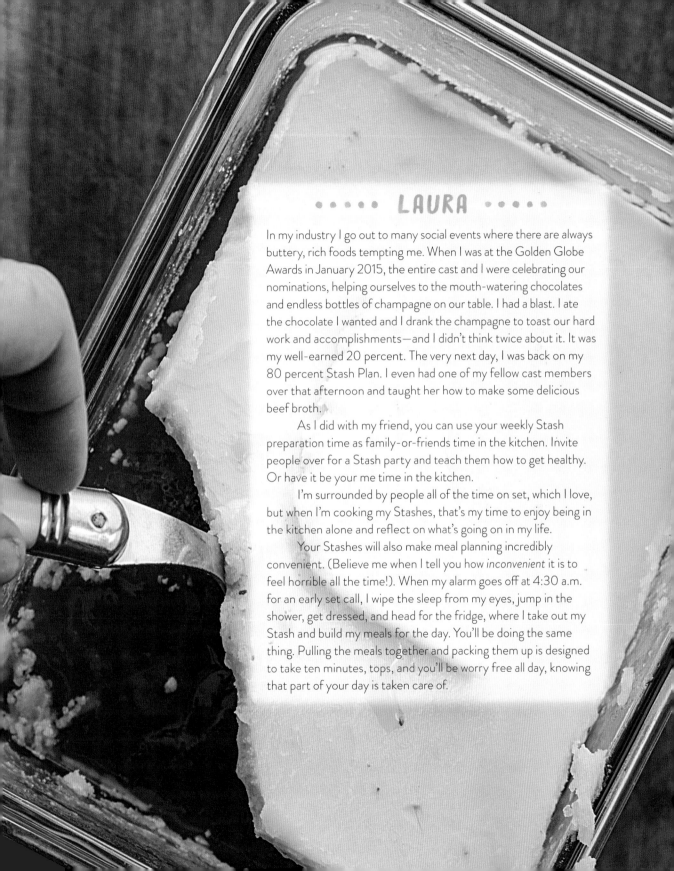

····· LAURA ·····

In my industry I go out to many social events where there are always buttery, rich foods tempting me. When I was at the Golden Globe Awards in January 2015, the entire cast and I were celebrating our nominations, helping ourselves to the mouth-watering chocolates and endless bottles of champagne on our table. I had a blast. I ate the chocolate I wanted and I drank the champagne to toast our hard work and accomplishments—and I didn't think twice about it. It was my well-earned 20 percent. The very next day, I was back on my 80 percent Stash Plan. I even had one of my fellow cast members over that afternoon and taught her how to make some delicious beef broth.

As I did with my friend, you can use your weekly Stash preparation time as family-or-friends time in the kitchen. Invite people over for a Stash party and teach them how to get healthy. Or have it be your me time in the kitchen.

I'm surrounded by people all of the time on set, which I love, but when I'm cooking my Stashes, that's my time to enjoy being in the kitchen alone and reflect on what's going on in my life.

Your Stashes will also make meal planning incredibly convenient. (Believe me when I tell you how *inconvenient* it is to feel horrible all the time!). When my alarm goes off at 4:30 a.m. for an early set call, I wipe the sleep from my eyes, jump in the shower, get dressed, and head for the fridge, where I take out my Stash and build my meals for the day. You'll be doing the same thing. Pulling the meals together and packing them up is designed to take ten minutes, tops, and you'll be worry free all day, knowing that part of your day is taken care of.

Why GOOD HEALTH starts FROM WITHIN

chapter 3

*In the chapters that follow, we are going to tell you
exactly what makes the Stash Plan so effective,
and how to eat and move to get the most benefit from
this program. But first it's important to give you
a little background information on why this method
works—and why other punishing, punitive
diet plans just don't (at least, not in the long term). It all
comes back to parts of our bodies that most of us don't
give a lot of thought to (until something goes terribly
wrong): your internal organs. Specifically,
your gallbladder and your liver.*

THE DYNAMIC DUO:
Your Gallbladder and Liver

THE GALLBLADDER AND LIVER are like an action-movie dynamic duo. They're the superhero cleansers and fat burners of your body. Just as Batman and Robin try to keep Gotham safe from a host of villains, so do the gallbladder and liver make our bodies safe from evil invaders. They strive to keep our metabolic function in harmony and our energy flowing smoothly. They also ensure that the evil invaders (the contaminants in our environment, the toxins we might eat, and the GMOs that have infiltrated our food chain) don't win. If, however, the evil invaders become too powerful and overwhelm the gallbladder and liver, these organs can't handle the onslaught. As you know already, this is what triggers a cascade of health problems.

The gallbladder and liver are utterly dependent on each other to function. They're a symbiotic pairing, working together to burn fat, create and store bile, and clean our blood, among many other processes detailed in this chapter.

When the liver is stressed, it stops metabolizing hormones, quits filtering blood properly, and won't give the gallbladder enough bile to do its job. When the gallbladder gets stressed, it shuts the floodgates and doesn't give the stored bile back to the liver, and this bile solidifies and crystallizes into gallstones. This robs you of your energy and makes you feel awful and gain weight.

We want these two superheroes to work efficiently to fight the evil henchmen, so here is the science you need to know to make sure this happens—and to ensure that you feel great!

What Your Gallbladder Does

Your gallbladder is located behind your liver on the right side of your rib cage. It is about the size of a dried apricot, but if it's not functioning well, it can puff up to the size of an avocado.

In Chinese Meridian Theory, as you may know, *all* energy starts in the gallbladder. The key is to get a great jump-start from the gallbladder to the liver—this is what triggers the healing and energizing process.

Your gallbladder and liver are codependent, because they are both involved in processing your food after you've eaten it. What links them is a substance called bile, which is produced in your liver.

The gallbladder is basically your body's storage reservoir for bile, a bitter (and if you've ever thrown up, you know what we're talking about), yellow fluid of vital importance for every person. Gallbladders are designed to hold over half the bile released from your liver, keeping it safe so that it's readily available in larger quantities whenever you eat.

• • • • • • • • • • • • **LAURA** • • • • • • • • • • • •

How many of us have been told by our parents, "Chew your food"? I always thought I chewed my food, but when I actually learned *why* chewing was so important, I really started paying close attention to it and realized that I was barely chewing at all. No wonder every time I ate my stomach was upset and my body was holding on to fat. No wonder I was hungry an hour after eating a big meal! My body thought it was starving because I wasn't actually assimilating the nutrients I was eating. We need to chew to help our bodies suck up these nutrients; it gives us more energy, we eat less, and we start burning fat. It may sound funny, but chewing was a game changer for me.

So the next time you eat a meal, sit at a table with no distractions and nobody talking to you. Give yourself twenty minutes to try this. I want you to chew every bite fifty times before swallowing. I'll bet you'll want to swallow after ten to fifteen chews, but keep going to fifty! When you get the food as broken down as it will be after the fiftieth chew, this is how every bite should be pulverized. You'll also realize how rushed we usually are while we're trying to eat. Chewing takes time! Once you start doing this, you'll realize how important it is to take this time for yourself. This food is what is powering your engine. Do your best to help your body get the nutrients you're giving it!

CLEAN BILE = HEALTH

Bile has two primary functions:

1. **Bile breaks down the fats in your food.** The salt in bile actually blends the difficult-to-digest fat in your food into a mixture that's easier for your small intestine to absorb and metabolize. This emulsification aids the digestive process, and it also neutralizes acids in partially digested food. That's why the better you chew your food, the easier it is to emulsify what you've just eaten, because you've already done a lot of the work breaking it into very small pieces with your teeth. You really *can't* chew your food too much. Think of it this way: Your stomach doesn't have teeth! You also need adequate bile in order to process the fat-soluble vitamins A, D, E, and K.

2. **Bile is a very powerful antioxidant**, which helps to remove harmful substances from the liver. (You'll learn a lot more about antioxidants in Chapter 6.) Part of the liver's job is to filter toxins out of your body, either via your bile ducts or directly into the small intestine.

The cleaner you can keep your bile, the more waste products can get filtered through and out of your body. These waste products are excreted primarily through your stool, as well as through urine and your skin. When we say "clean bile," what we mean is that it's flowing smoothly, able to break down and emulsify toxins so that when there is a foreign invader, it can handle it. The fewer environmental toxins you are exposed to and the purer the food you eat, the cleaner your bile.

In addition, the cleaner your bile, the more easily it can break down fats during digestion. If, however, you eat processed food with GMOs and your body is constantly bombarded with toxins, your bile production slows down. The bile you have gets sludgy and sluggish.

This is how gallstones are created. When the bile is stuck, it doesn't move—instead, its salts crystallize and start to clump together. Gallstones can be formed very easily, and most people don't even know that they have them. Usually gallstones become noticeable only when you start to have some or all of the same kinds of health problems Laura did: low energy, stomach pains, and an overall feeling of being unwell.

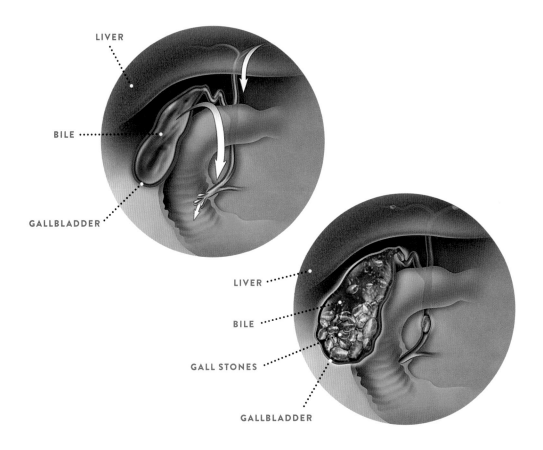

LIVER

BILE

GALLBLADDER

LIVER

BILE

GALL STONES

GALLBLADDER

The easiest way to visualize what your gallbladder does is to think of it as your body's trusty garbage truck, making the rounds every day. If the garbage in the back of the truck doesn't get regularly dumped, you can't cram any more garbage into it or it just gets stuck. If your gallbladder can't get properly flushed of all the bile and toxins it's storing, this directly affects your liver, which then gets sluggish, too. And when this happens, your stressed-out gallbladder can no longer handle all those toxins we ingest on a regular basis, whether we've eaten them, drunk them, or inhaled them. There's no way for all of those toxins to be eliminated—which means that your fat-burning, your metabolism, and your normal hormone regulation all slow down. It's like you're trying to walk through two feet of muck in a swamp. Nobody wants that!

What Your Liver Does

Your liver is located in the upper right portion of the abdominal cavity, under the diaphragm, and weighs three to four pounds. It is a vital organ that supports nearly every other organ in your body in some facet. Without a healthy liver, you cannot survive.

Bile, which we discussed in the previous section, helps to digest the fat in your diet. The bile is stored in your gallbladder, but it is actually created in your liver, which is why the health of your liver and the health of your gallbladder are so closely intertwined. Holy matrimony, in sickness and in health, as long as they both shall live.

The liver truly is a kick-ass organ, with multiple functions:

1. **The liver is your body's filter, the largest detoxing organ you have.** And it's on call every second of every minute of every hour of every day. Your liver processes everything you eat, drink, breathe in, or rub on your skin. It's like having a built-in chemical processing factory, neutralizing the harmful things you take in on a daily basis.

   As your body's filter, the liver has to decipher what you've ingested any time you eat or drink. Is it a chemical? Is it a foreign substance? Is it potentially toxic? Is it a recognizable food needed by your body and easily digestible?

   When your liver doesn't recognize something you've ingested—a GMO-laden piece of food, for example—it is classified as a foreign substance. We like to call these foreign substances "evil invaders," because that's what they are! Since your body is always on alert to stay alive and protect you from evil invaders, it stores these toxic substances either in your fat or in the liver itself. It does this to keep all your other sensitive vital organs safe.

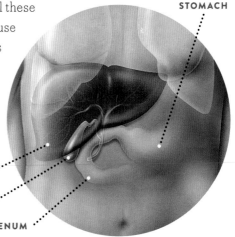

STOMACH

LIVER

GALLBLADDER

DUODENUM

It might be annoying to have cellulite, but your body thinks it is *helping* you by stuffing the toxins there. So let's help your liver get rid of these evil invaders so they're no longer stored in unwanted dimples on your booty!

2. **The liver is the Laundromat for your blood,** filtering out harmful chemicals that enter your bloodstream and cleansing the blood of wastes. It also allows more blood into circulation when needed.

3. **The liver filters hormones from our bodies.** Of course a healthy body produces hormones, and that's exactly what it should be doing. But increasingly, we're ingesting hormones via the food we eat, and this is where our livers can get overwhelmed. This happens when, for example, cows are pumped full of hormones to produce milk faster, or steers are pumped full of hormones in order to mature faster and "beef up" so they weigh more (which translates to higher profits for the farmers). When you drink the tainted milk or meat or by-products from such animals, you are ingesting whatever was given to them, too.

   Much research has been published on the alarming rise of precocious puberty. According to a study conducted by researchers from the University of Brighton and published in the journal *Public Health Nutrition* in 2010, young girls who eat a diet higher in meat reach puberty significantly earlier than girls who eat less meat. Dr. Joseph Mercola, a well-known proponent of alternative medicine and an osteopathic physician, has stated that "the primary reason why diet may be a driving factor behind the early puberty phenomenon is the excessive use of hormones and other estrogen-mimicking chemicals in livestock and dairy production."

   In addition, if the liver becomes overwhelmed by the amount of hormonal activity, and it isn't being given the proper nutrients it needs to help process toxins, it can't work at top capacity. Unwanted hormones and toxins can then wreak havoc in other areas of the body.

4. **The liver is a major part of the digestive process.** After you eat, your liver allows small particles of nutrients to pass through the upper part of the small intestine, called the duodenum. The duodenum collects the bile produced by the liver and absorbs the small particles of nutrients broken down by the bile.

5. **The liver is the only organ that can regenerate itself.** Amazing, isn't it? Dr. George Michalopoulos, professor and chairman of the Department of Pathology at the University of Pittsburgh, explains that "liver regeneration is very complex and a well-orchestrated phenomenon. The liver manages to restore any lost mass, while at the same time providing full support for the body." What's even more amazing is that the Stash Plan helps you to revamp and reenergize your liver function again. You will have clean bile and fresh new blood. And a perfectly functioning gallbladder that enhances liver functioning, too.

Meridian Fundamentals

NOW THAT YOU HAVE THE SKINNY on what the liver and gallbladder do, let's talk about what meridians are, how they correlate to energy, and why they're so vital to the functioning of not just these two organs but your entire body. We love demystifying wisdom of the ages!

Meridians were discovered by ancient masters practicing meditation, qigong, yoga, and other types of holistic mind-body work. These masters trained to immerse themselves deeply in another state of consciousness and literally learned to see inside the body and alter its energy pathways. This is called invisible energy work.

There's nothing woo-woo about invisible energy work. So much of what we use and don't even bother to think about every minute of every day is invisible—solar radiation, light, airwaves, electricity, gravity, sonar, Wi-Fi . . . even your thoughts, knowledge, and love itself. Accepting this invisible energy means you're opening yourself to all the power of your qi.

A meridian is a predictable electrical pathway of energy in all life-forms; it's a collection of points woven into a web by lines of travel. These pathways are identical in every person. They are invisible and connect to every atom, cell, tendon, ligament, and bone; to every millimeter of your skin; to all your brain cells; and much more! It's believed that meridians are fired by electrical impulses that go through water; and we, as humans, are comprised of approximately 75 percent water.

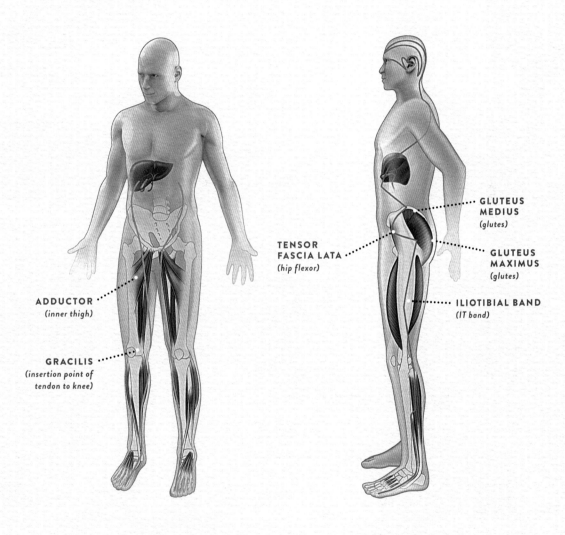

**TENSOR
FASCIA LATA**
(hip flexor)

**GLUTEUS
MEDIUS**
(glutes)

**GLUTEUS
MAXIMUS**
(glutes)

ADDUCTOR
(inner thigh)

ILIOTIBIAL BAND
(IT band)

GRACILIS
*(insertion point of
tendon to knee)*

LIVER MERIDIAN

GALLBLADDER MERIDIAN

Think of it this way: If you see a live wire lying on your street after a thunderstorm brought it down, the last place you want to be is in a nearby puddle of water. Why? Because if this wire was to hit the water, the electricity would shoot through it and you'd get a pretty hefty zap. It's the same reason why your parents wouldn't let you swim in the swimming pool during a lightning storm.

This invisible energy (qi) travels along these meridians just like a train on its tracks. Each of these meridians is correlated to a specific organ. For example, to bring more energy to the gallbladder and liver, you can do very specific things to "fire" these specific meridians—which is what the Stash Plan is all about.

Firing a meridian means that energy is moving through a specific line or pathway and creating more vibrations in the organ correlated to that pathway. This flow follows a predictable pattern; certain stops are trigger points. When you activate those points, whether through food or stretching, the whole meridian is fired. Energy flow is released and the functioning of the correlated organ starts to improve.

Jon Gabriel, author of *The Gabriel Method*, explains, "Chinese medicine believes that stress, toxins, low-energy thinking, and negative emotions cause blockages in the flow of subtle energy, and that these blockages are the root of all sickness and depression . . . blocked energy stagnates, and stagnation is devitalization. Just as a stagnant puddle of water is less healthy to drink than a flowing stream, the stagnant energy in our bodies is less healthy than flowing energy."

When traffic is moving smoothly along your meridians, your qi is flowing through as it should be as if you're cruising down the road while listening to your favorite tunes. A blockage to your meridians due to tight muscles and fascia buildup is like that same freeway during the height of rush hour: Bottlenecked cars are trying to merge into this already packed freeway with nowhere to go, creeping along, or worse . . . stopped entirely.

You can fire your meridians in many ways: acupuncture, acupressure, movement (particularly the kind of targeted stretching you'll learn about in this book), intense emotions, and of course, eating the right kind of food. In particular, the Stash Plan kind of food. Getting your gallbladder and liver to function at their highest capacity is the crux of the Stash Plan.

WHAT HAPPENS WHEN YOUR
Gallbladder and Liver Aren't Functioning Correctly?

YOU KNOW THOSE SCENES in action movies where all the evil hench-men suddenly surround the superhero, and you wonder how Batman and Robin are going to outwit the machinations of the Joker or the Penguin? Sometimes there are so many diabolical henchmen that the dynamic duo is overwhelmed and spirited back to the evil nemesis's lair. There the super-heroes use their superior wits and strength to fight the bad guys and sur-vive to tell the tale—and of course make a sequel!

It's the same thing with our superheroes, the gallbladder and liver, the Digestive Duo. When the evil invaders in the form of the unrecogniz-able foreign substances you've ingested overwhelm them, they get *stuck*. The liver can no longer do its job purifying your blood and burning fat and filtering out toxins; these toxins can escape via the blood and collect around the joints, worsening arthritis or wreaking havoc in other parts of the body. The gallbladder can no longer give the liver the bile it needs to do its job. Everything backs up and slows down. This dynamic duo becomes about as thrilling as volcanic lava inching its way down a mountain, collect-ing a ton of debris and detritus along the way. All that accumulated stuff makes even burning hot lava sludgy—exactly what happens to your bile, too.

This is a serious problem, as people eating a typical American diet put food in their mouth on average three to six times a day. Bile is released every time—but more and more bile is needed to break down the kinds of processed, GMO-laden foods many of us unwittingly consume, and those very foods make that bile sludgy and less effective (just when your body needs it the most). It's a vicious circle.

Many things can go awry when your gallbladder and liver are not functioning correctly:

- **Fat-burning stops.** A liver that's stuck can't metabolize fat properly. Unused fat can't go anywhere—your body is programmed to hold on to it in the form of fat cells. Which are in turn stored all over your body—making you gain weight!

- **At the same time, your appetite increases,** because you're not getting the proper nutrients your body desperately needs.

- **The liver can't aid in the digestive process properly,** to help break down food. Bile's two jobs, as you read earlier in this chapter, are to carry waste away and to break down fats during digestion. When the evil invaders overwhelm your gallbladder and liver, however, the bile gets backed up and waste isn't eliminated, as it should be.

- **Toxins go into your lymphatic system,** which is your internal immune system. You'll learn more about it on page 89 in Chapter 4. For now, know that, unlike your circulatory system carrying blood around your body, the system is not bound by vessels or arteries; it is free-flowing. This is crucial for survival. Whenever there is a foreign invader in the body, lymphocytes, or natural killer cells, are able to travel there and fight infection. The lymph nodes' job is to absorb these pathogens and kill them. However, when the lymph nodes become too full of toxins, they can't take in any more invaders. The red velvet rope goes up; the venue is at full capacity; the pathogens go find someplace else to cause a ruckus. People with a "stuck" liver and gallbladder get sick more often than others, because their bodies are already stressed and overloaded.

  Your lymphatic system can also become sluggish when bile gets stuck; if the movement of waste out of your body gets clogged due to this stuck bile, it becomes more difficult to remove fluid. You retain water and can become extremely bloated. Nobody likes that. Especially Laura when she has to fit into her wardrobe for camera.

- **You have "brain fog,"** a cloudy, almost dopey feeling that makes it hard to concentrate. This is caused by a lack of good nutrition, dehydration, and too many toxins, such as heavy metals, pesticides, and pollutants. Isaac Eliaz of *Rodale News* explains it this way: "Nutrition affects every system in the body, but especially the brain. Traditional Chinese Medicine, for example, has long associated cognitive power with strong digestion. . . . Junk foods high in sugars and trans fats fuel inflammation and impair cognitive function. Worse, insulin dysfunction—usually related to chronically elevated blood sugar from an unhealthy diet—is a major risk factor in dementia and cognitive decline." In addition, molecules called free radicals (which you'll learn about in Chapter 6) can lower long-term cognitive function over time. Good thing the food you'll be eating on the Stash Plan helps rid you of brain fog!

- **You have indigestion.** This is due to the bile being acidic. The gallbladder dumps more and more bile into the liver while trying to help its partner break down whatever we've ingested. It's trying to bring firepower to the liver to fight off the evil invaders.

- **You get very constipated** with a low-functioning gallbladder and liver. Without adequate bile production, food is not digested properly, leading to a lack of lubrication in the large intestine.

- **You can develop allergies.** These are often the result of an overloaded toxic state within the liver. As you now know, the liver is our filter and chemical processing plant, but if the number of evil invaders is too high, the immune system rushes to the aid. It classifies the evil invaders as allergens and produces antibodies to fight them off. We believe this is one of the reasons why clinical diagnoses of allergies have soared dramatically in the last few decades. As Dr. Mercola explains: "At an alarming rate, people's immune systems are overreacting to substances that should be harmless, leading to allergies; in others, their immune systems are malfunctioning and attacking parts of their own body—the very definition of autoimmune disease." You may recognize some of these autoimmune disorders as celiac disease, diabetes,

LAURA

· · · · ·

One of the many doctors I consulted diagnosed me with Hashimoto's thyroiditis, an autoimmune disorder of the thyroid, the gland in your neck that produces hormones coordinating many of your body's activities. I found out that a common occurrence with this syndrome is that every time I ate gluten, my immune system was so confused and malfunctioning that it thought gluten was trying to attack me and sent out antibodies that would attack my very own thyroid. While I have followed the Stash Plan, my symptoms have drastically reduced, and my blood work has since shown normal levels of thyroid functioning. Which is a huge relief!

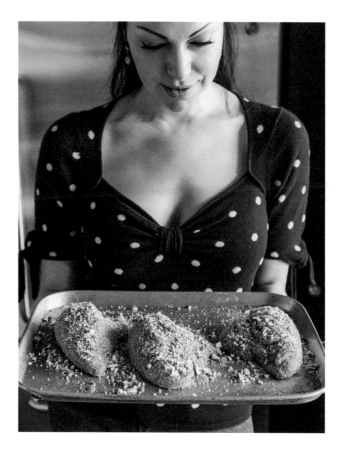

Sjögren's syndrome, rheumatoid arthritis, Hashimoto's thyroiditis, and Graves' disease, just to name a few.

- **You get headaches.** The number one pattern underlying migraines is the stagnation of energy flow to the liver. Liver-related headaches tend to run along the temples because the gallbladder meridian—which is closely connected to the liver—travels through this area as well.

- **You have a variety of skin problems.** Your skin, as you know, is your body's largest organ, and the release or buildup of impurities or toxins often causes acne, blotchiness, boils, dryness, eczema, and an overall dullness. There is not enough makeup or zit cream to cover up the effects of a gallbladder and liver that aren't doing their jobs properly.

GALLBLADDERS AND LIVERS ARE IMPAIRED BY . . .

- Antibiotics
- Arsenic, commonly found in fluoride, processed wood such as particleboard, and some cosmetics
- Chlorine-bleached products, such as tampons
- Cigarette smoke
- Dry-cleaning plastic and chemicals. Fortunately, organic dry cleaners are becoming more prevalent.
- Environmental toxins, such as pollutants in the air like car exhaust and the burning of fossil fuels
- Fluoride-enhanced and chlorinated tap water. Fluoride might be great at cavity prevention but it is highly toxic, and as such, it is often used in pesticides and rodenticides.
- Painkillers
- Pesticides and herbicides
- Preservatives
- Processing plants
- Tea bags, unless they're organic. The bleach used to make tea bags white seeps into the tea leaves. This is also the case with coffee filters.
- Preservatives

WHAT IS A TOXIN?

What does it really mean to detox? A toxin is a poison or an unhealthy/bad substance that can cause you harm. Detoxing means you're removing the toxins from the blood in the liver (which as you now know is your blood's washing machine), eliminating toxins through intestines, kidneys, and skin, as well as refueling your body with the right kind of food.

Toxins have many different ways of manifesting in your body.

Sometimes, for example, you might have a coated white tongue, especially in the morning, due to toxins coming from the liver. Think of your tongue as a compost pile where the fumes sit on top. When you breathe while you're sleeping, your tongue catches all the fumes and saliva and keeps them on top.

Eczema, pimples, acne, and rashes are all signs of toxins coming out through your skin.

Cellulite, in fact, is caused by toxins trapped in fat cells or lymph nodes, which gives it that dimpled appearance; even rail-thin supermodels can have dimpled booties. (That's why liposuction can remove fat cells but cannot fully remove cellulite.)

All those things with a certain odor that you dread having—halitosis, or bad breath; smelly farts; and potent body odor—can be caused by toxins.

But even if you don't smell, don't have bad breath, aren't gassy, and are free of cellulite, you can still be loaded with toxins. These are all signs you might have toxin overload:

LAURA

• • • • • • •

When I go to industry functions or parties in Hollywood, what are the typical topics of conversation? Directors, producers, casting—and the latest detox cleanses. Juice cleanses, master cleanses, soup cleanses, fruit cleanses, no sugar/no grains cleanses, cleanses involving nothing but water and appetite suppressants, just to name a few. All meant to "detox" the body.

- General fatigue

- Sleep issues (insomnia, restless sleep)

- An inability to lose weight, even though you're exercising regularly and cutting back calories

- Constipation

- A sensitivity to smoke, chemicals, or fumes in the environment

- Thirst (drinking less than sixty-four daily ounces of untainted water)

- Itchy, burning eyes or blurred vision

- Recurring sinus problems, such as postnasal drip

- Slow-growing hair and nails

- Thinning hair

- Nonspecific aches and pains

These aren't just symptoms of "getting older" or being stressed. These are signs of toxins.

ELIZABETH

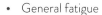

I often see and feel the aftereffects of toxicity when my clients come with hangovers to my classes on Sunday morning. They can't stretch like they normally would in a class during the week. Why? Because in Chinese Meridian Theory, the body parts associated with the liver are your tendons. So if their livers are in overdrive trying to handle the booze from the previous night, they could pull a tendon in class. I have to walk on them twice as long to flush these toxins out first, before they can even start to stretch. When most people think of tendons, they think of their knees and elbows. However, your body has tendons everywhere. A nifty li'l fact is that there are tendons attached to the back of the eyes to keep them in place. One of the reasons you get blurred vision when you're drinking too much is due to the alcohol's effect on the liver, which in turn affects the tendons.

The Stash Plan is designed to slowly flush the toxins out of your body, with its healthy eating plan containing food and drink with no GMOs or other unnatural chemicals and preservatives. Your energy increases, you lose weight, your skin is clearer, you sleep better, and aches and pains gradually disappear.

Common Illnesses/Conditions of the Gallbladder

A common gallbladder problem is gallstones. Without regular dumping, stored bile can crystallize into small, hard deposits inside the gallbladder, especially when the bile salts and cholesterol that are the essential components of bile itself fall out of balance with each other (often due to high cholesterol levels). This is one of the reasons your gallbladder can puff up to the size of an avocado. We love avocados, but not in *this* context!

OUR *bodies* **ARE VERY** *smart.*

According to a study done by Dr. Ronald Hoffman of the Albert Einstein College of Medicine in 2013, "Up to 20 million Americans have undiagnosed gallbladder disease." This is the inability for the gallbladder to break down and remove gallstones. This seems like a pretty large figure for a condition that can often be eradicated by doing the Stash Plan.

Another study by Dr. Hoffman published in 2013 showed that in Saudi Arabia, gallbladder disease has increased by an astonishing *600 percent* since they began eating a mostly Western diet in the late 1960s. His theory is that there is a significant correlation between high-sugar and processed foods and gallbladder malfunction.

Common Illnesses/Conditions of the Liver

One of the most well-known liver diseases is cirrhosis, which is often caused by excessive alcohol consumption and involves healthy liver tissue being replaced by scar tissue. Eating processed, nonorganic food can cause cirrhosis as well, in part because the bile ducts can get clogged; and because pesticide- and preservative-laced and genetically modified food makes your body acidic without your even drinking a drop of alcohol.

Another serious liver condition is fatty liver disease, which is triggered when fat accumulates in the liver, causing scarring and inflammation. These scars also block bile ducts and blood circulation throughout the liver.

It has been thought that fatty liver is primarily caused by either alcohol abuse or obesity. However, one theory is that this is also caused by bad and denatured foods laden with GMOs, pesticides, and herbicides. Why? Because when the liver is overwhelmed by environmental toxins ingested due to an unhealthy diet, it becomes unable to metabolize fat properly and stores it inside itself instead, in its own fat cells.

Crash diets can also cause fatty liver, because they trick your body into thinking it is in starvation mode. When this happens, the liver accumulates fat inside itself in order to keep functioning, because if your body thinks it's starving, it will hold on to *any* fat so that it can survive. This would unwittingly happen to Laura every time she would put herself on a torturous crash diet. Consuming a diet with a healthy balance of natural fats actually prevents fatty liver.

Our bodies are very smart; they are always looking to survive to their highest potential. When we ingest foreign or toxic substances, our bodies need to figure out where to put them. Normally, it's the liver's job as the body's chemical filtration system to handle them. However, when it is overtaxed, the liver basically gives up and either keeps these substances inside itself or sends it to be stored in fat cells in other areas of the body. Your body uses fat as a cushion, literally and figuratively, to protect you from harm from within and without. Rid yourself of the need for this protective fat and you are on your way to ridding yourself of a fatty liver.

HOW STRESS AFFECTS
Your Gallbladder and Liver

THE EVERYDAY STRESSES OF MODERN LIFE can wreak havoc on your gallbladder and liver, too.

- **Sitting is killer.** Many of us spend endless hours at our desks, in our offices, staring at a computer screen for much of the day. Then we sit in a car or a bus or a train to get home. The gallbladder meridian runs up through the hip flexor (in the front of your hip), and the primary trigger point for this meridian is in the gluteus muscles of your booty. The liver meridian runs up the inside of your legs. When these meridians are constricted and blocked due to constant sitting and lack of movement, their functioning is severely affected.

Following the Stash Plan, especially the stretches, will keep these meridians open. While you are in the office at the computer, take a short break and do a stretch whenever possible. Each stretch takes only a few minutes; you can intersperse them throughout the day or do them in the morning or at night. A few minutes is all you need to unblock the stuck energy—believe us, you'll feel a difference right away.

- **Eating processed food stresses your body.** As you've already learned (and will read much more about in the next chapter), your liver can't recognize a processed food as a real food, even if it's had nutrients such as vitamins and minerals added to it. Artificial sweeteners, artificial fillers, artificial colors, fake food, preservatives, and GMOs are all evil invaders. So are low-calorie diets filled with processed food; diet or so-called energy bars; fat-free yogurts loaded with sugar-drenched fruit; baked goods where the fat is replaced with sugar; and fake foods such as diet margarine and whipped toppings like Cool Whip.

- **Hectic schedules affect the gallbladder and liver as well.** When Laura gets up for five a.m. call times and works seventeen-hour days, she needs to find a balance so that her body doesn't give up on her—but that became impossible when she was so lacking in energy.

  When your body gets stressed, especially by something sudden—a pedestrian's darting out in front of your car; hearing a loud and unexpected noise; your boss's constantly yelling—or just daily stress from work or family as well as emotional stress from a partner, this triggers the release of stress hormones, primarily cortisol and adrenaline. These are hormones that are released by the hypothalamus, a part of the brain at the back of the head

  The word *hypothalamus* comes from the Greek words meaning under and room. Its function is to collect and combine data and send signals to fix any imbalances, from regulating body temperature and blood pressure, telling your body you're hungry or full, and managing the stress hormones to prime your body for the fight-or-flight mode. This basically is your body's survival mechanism, an evolutionary remnant of the cave-dweller era, when dangers were constant and bodies needed to be ready to hurry to safety with barely a moment's notice.

LAURA

A friend of mine who worked on a game reserve in South Africa told me a story that blew me away. At night they would set up fences protecting the area around the group of people camping. They would shine large lights out into the brush to spot any lions that might be in the vicinity. One night, after the fence work was done, my friend was patrolling, and out of nowhere in the blink of an eye, a lion stealthily approached the fence, ready to pounce. My friend told me that he literally jumped up and back what felt like twenty feet, away from that lion, back to safety. It was one of those moments of superhuman strength—his fight-or-flight mode saving his hide.

We might now be living in the digital age, but our bodies still have the same internal functioning of our ancestors from a long time ago. We might not be fighting off mastodons and saber-toothed tigers, but we are fighting off daily stresses. The constant hormonal surges that result are not good for us. Long-term levels of increased cortisol can lead to impaired cognitive and thyroid functions, anxiety and depression, increased fatigue and insomnia, blood sugar imbalances, digestive issues, high blood pressure, decreased muscle tissue and bone density, lowered immunity and inflammatory responses, and increased deposits of abdominal fat.

When I started working on healing my gallbladder and liver, I realized my stressful lifestyle kept me in chronic fight-or-flight mode just to get through every day. I was in absolute adrenaline and cortisol overload, and the result of this oversaturation of stress hormones paradoxically made me more tired, not energized at all. I loved my life . . . so why was my body telling me that I was in danger every moment of the day? I knew that I needed to find a solution for this.

This situation is very common for those dealing with daily stress and pressure. When I learned to eat to support my gallbladder and liver and do my daily stretches, my body calmed down and my stress hormones returned to normal levels.

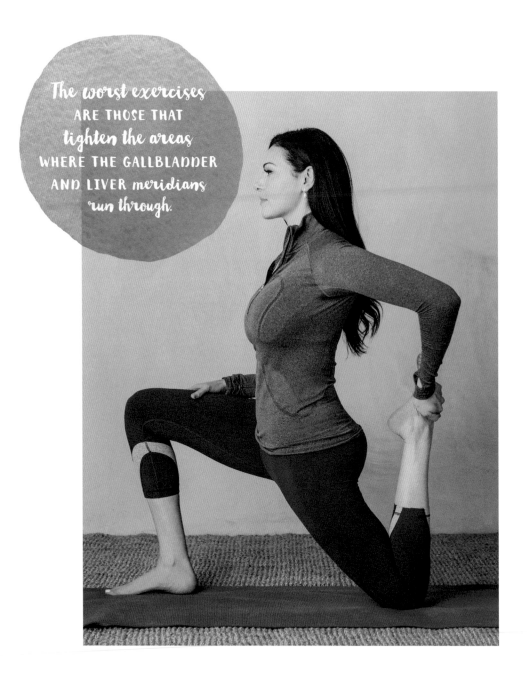

The worst exercises ARE THOSE THAT tighten the areas WHERE THE GALLBLADDER AND LIVER meridians run through.

Get Fit or Get Fat: THE BEST (AND WORST) EXERCISES FOR YOUR GALLBLADDER AND LIVER

Do These Exercises to Support the Stash Plan

The exercises with the best effect on your gallbladder and liver are those that open and create an energy flow through the gallbladder and liver meridians. These are exercises that do not make your hip flexors and glutes tight in the area where the gallbladder and liver meridians flow. You always want to keep these areas unaffected and open when you work out.

We recommend the following exercises instead:

- **Bike riding.** Avoid bikes with downward-facing handlebars, such as racing bikes. Instead, choose an upright cruiser, as it keeps your torso elevated and allows for easy movement of the hip flexors and glutes.

- **Dancing.** All kinds of dance are great for the gallbladder and liver, whether it's hitting a club or taking Argentine tango lessons, like Laura loves to do. Dancing gives us a sense of freedom and creative physical expression.

- **Power walking.** Striding upright and extending your hip flexors and quadriceps (front thigh muscles) helps propel you forward. Swinging your arms also stimulates the gallbladder and liver meridians running through your upper body.

- **Racquetball and squash.** These sports involve constant use of the gallbladder/liver muscle groups in the upper and lower body, especially the glutes and the lats.

- **Rebounding.** Jumping on a small trampoline, or rebounding, stimulates the peristalsis (involuntary muscle movement) in the gallbladder to allow bile to release when it should. Rebounding also helps to circulate more blood in and out of the liver as well as flush out lymphatic fluid.

- **Rowing, especially on open water.** This all-body exercise uses the lats as well as the glutes and the IT band when you push off with your legs and pull back with your arms and shoulders.

- **Running.** This activity is especially good at helping gallbladders flush out bile. Outdoor runs are better than indoor runs on treadmills; the fresh air on your skin is more invigorating and stimulating.

- **Skiing.** The side-to-side bouncing motion (especially if you do moguls) on skis engages your lats, glutes, and IT bands.

Avoid These Exercises on the Stash Plan . . . at Least in the Beginning

The worst exercises are those that tighten the areas where the gallbladder and liver meridians run through. They might ostensibly be good for your cardiovascular health or for muscle strengthening, but they can paradoxically leave you feeling sluggish, not energized. However, once you learn how to do the Stash stretches and do them every day, these exercises can gradually be reintroduced as part of your regular workouts.

- **Pilates.** Many people like the idea that Pilates strengthens your core. When the "core" is referred to, you're actually talking about the psoas muscle. This muscle connects the lumbar spine to the hip flexor to the pelvis. It moves from the front of the body up to the back. But when the psoas or core is constricted, it blocks energy from being able to travel to the gallbladder and liver. Precisely what you don't want!

- **Stair steppers.** They not only tighten your hip flexors, thus affecting the gallbladder meridian, but also block the liver meridian and impede the flow of bile into the liver.

- **Squats.** When you do squats, you shorten and tighten your hip flexors and glutes, and you contract and shorten your quads. Not to mention that they wreak havoc on your knees.

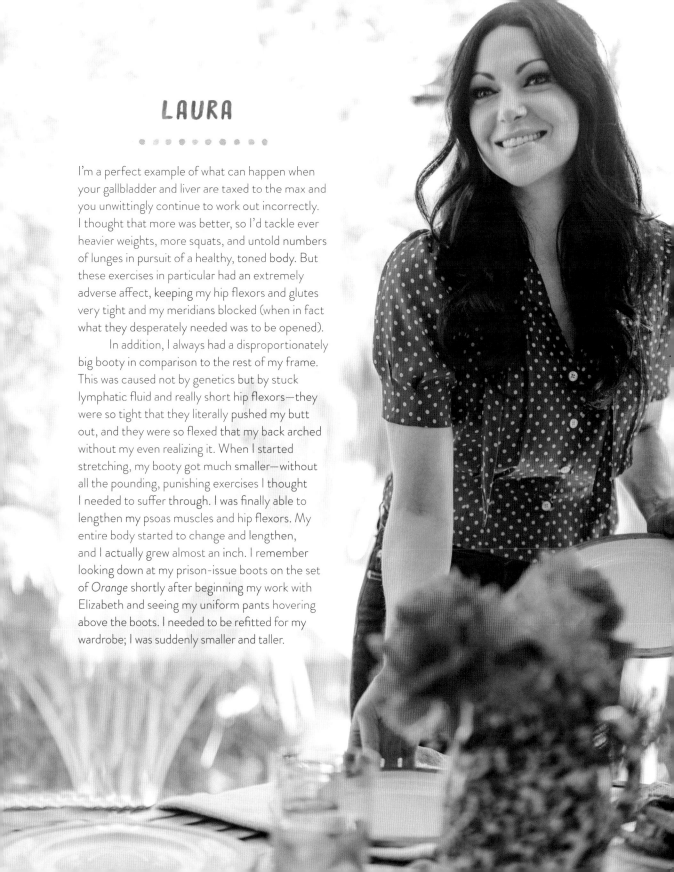

LAURA

I'm a perfect example of what can happen when your gallbladder and liver are taxed to the max and you unwittingly continue to work out incorrectly. I thought that more was better, so I'd tackle ever heavier weights, more squats, and untold numbers of lunges in pursuit of a healthy, toned body. But these exercises in particular had an extremely adverse affect, keeping my hip flexors and glutes very tight and my meridians blocked (when in fact what they desperately needed was to be opened).

In addition, I always had a disproportionately big booty in comparison to the rest of my frame. This was caused not by genetics but by stuck lymphatic fluid and really short hip flexors—they were so tight that they literally pushed my butt out, and they were so flexed that my back arched without my even realizing it. When I started stretching, my booty got much smaller—without all the pounding, punishing exercises I thought I needed to suffer through. I was finally able to lengthen my psoas muscles and hip flexors. My entire body started to change and lengthen, and I actually grew almost an inch. I remember looking down at my prison-issue boots on the set of *Orange* shortly after beginning my work with Elizabeth and seeing my uniform pants hovering above the boots. I needed to be refitted for my wardrobe; I was suddenly smaller and taller.

How to FUEL YOUR Lean Mean SEXY MACHINE

chapter 4

Put regular gas in a precision, high-performance Lamborghini, and you'll never get it to perform properly. Put the regular sugar-laden, chemical-drenched, genetically modified food of the typical American diet in your body . . . and good luck feeling your best.

High-performance vehicles like our bodies need high-performance fuel. And it's really easy to get it once you know how to eat.

Comparing our bodies to race cars is an apt analogy because, after all, our bodies are beautiful machines. They are built in a skillful way to perform all the amazing tasks necessary to keep us functioning, while powering the mechanisms that make us stay alive as thinking and feeling beings.

The Stash Plan is akin to a pit stop on a racetrack. This is the home base for the race car, where the car gets gassed up, tires and wheels are checked, the oil is changed, and the parts tuned up and tweaked before it's sent back out into the race. Of course we Americans as a culture are *always* racing, and our bodies are trying to keep up. Our bodies are constantly striving to do their best while having to deal with ordinary workday stress, the processing of environmental toxins and GMOs, and the necessity to balance the needs of our families and friends.

But they need help. They need premium fuel (in the form of the best possible food) and constant maintenance (in the form of regular stretching, exercise, and stress relief). Wouldn't it be amazing to have our very own pit stop, a place where we could get fine-tuned and tinkered with before having to head back out to the race, so we can function at our highest capacity? With the Stash Plan you can have just that.

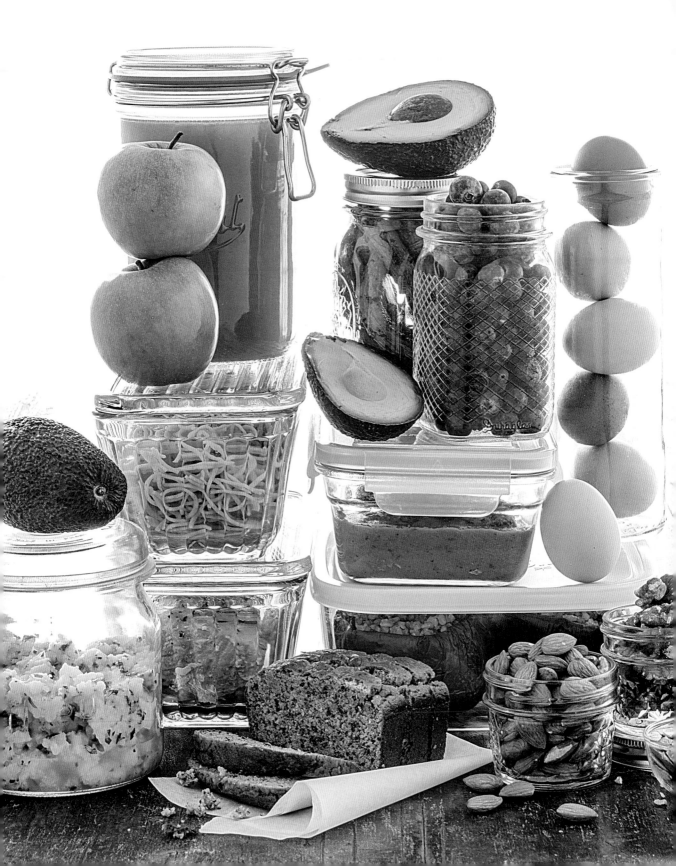

This is what you need for the marvelous machine that is your body:

- **The fuel:** unprocessed, GMO-free, organic, pure Stash Plan food.

- **The machine parts:** stretches to keep the nuts and bolts tightened and working efficiently the way they are supposed to.

- **The oil:** homemade broth to lubricate our bodies while its micronutrients heal us at a systemic level.

- **The combustion:** energy flowing through our meridians smoothly, without any blockage or impediment.

Fuel is the predominant component of the Stash Plan. You need fuel in the form of food to function. And the right kind of fuel is crucial. The wrong kind can literally leave you running on empty—or worse, stalling out. And we know that's not an option for you!

Sometimes we hear people say, "Oh, I know I have weight problems and health problems—it's because of my genes. My family's genetic history is just terrible." That can be true, of course. But might it be possible that their family history of health problems has been caused by a family history of eating fast food and processed junk food five days a week? Eating the right kinds of food from the Stash Plan helps to optimize your genetic potential.

How Our Modern Diet and GMOs
STRESS YOUR GALLBLADDER AND LIVER

THE FUEL WE NEED to power our machines must be wholesome, as unprocessed as possible, and untainted by chemicals or anything that can possibly be toxic. Remember, the liver has to be able to recognize this fuel as full of genuine nutrients so it can be processed and metabolized properly. As you already know, the liver is your body's chemical processing plant. Every single substance you ingest is filtered through the liver—good, nutritious food or unhealthy stuff like GMOs (or genetically modified organisms), pesticides, herbicides, and environmental toxins. A liver that is constantly bombarded with evil invaders needs a lot of firepower and emergency assistance to ward off these bad guys.

This fuel needs to be grown in rich soil without any external toxins such as pesticides or herbicides; be free of any taint from GMO ingredients; or, if it's from an animal source, raised on diets without GMOs or hormones.

The Origin of Packaged Foods and GMOs

In 1908, a Japanese researcher isolated a new taste substance from the seaweed called kombu. He noted it had a taste very different from sweet, sour, bitter, or salty. He called that taste *umami*. This substance was chemically replicated a year later.

Chemically speaking, MSG, short for monosodium glutamate, is 78 percent free glutamic acid, 21 percent sodium, and up to 1 percent contaminants. Free glutamic acid is the *same* neurotransmitter that your brain, nervous system, eyes, pancreas, and liver use to initiate processes in your body. Your body actually knows how to naturally produce glutamic acid, so if more of it is artificially introduced, this creates a spiraling effect of miscommunication in your nervous system. MSG is an excitotoxin, which means it overexcites your cells to the point of damage or death.

MSG began to be sold as a food additive. Fast-forward a few decades, to the post–World War II years, when canned soups, stews, spaghetti, and TV dinners began to be manufactured—and sold to the public as "healthy." MSG was an inexpensive way to make this type of food extra-palatable, even though through processing and the preservation process, the food had been stripped of many of its nutrients and its taste. MSG is a wholly fake, make-believe flavor enhancer, and consumers were fooled into thinking they were eating nutritious food because it tasted good. Why wouldn't they be? Packaged foods were a revelation when they hit the market. They were convenient, they were inexpensive, and kids really loved them. Parents

IF YOU DON'T *recognize* AN INGREDIENT, YOUR *body* WON'T EITHER.

(mostly moms, in that era) who'd previously spent hours shopping and cooking relished the ease of preparation with these new foods.

Yet all these people were duped. They thought they were buying premium fuel for their engines when they were actually getting the cheapest watered-down economy gasoline, which was slowly but steadily eroding them from the inside out. Worse, MSG is not quite the benign additive many have touted it to be for decades. There is a tremendous amount of anecdotal evidence reporting that the glutamate component of MSG is a neurotoxin and as such poses a risk for neurological damage and cancer. This is because glutamate levels tend to be high in cancer patients, as reported by a well-known study published in *International Immunology* in 1991. Even the FDA admits that MSG is what they classify as a GRAS (generally recognized as safe) additive—largely because so many adverse reactions to MSG have been reported over the years that it can't be considered wholly benign. That's like saying, have four drinks, then drive, and "generally" you'll make it home in one piece.

As the years went by, the number of packaged foods increased dramatically, which meant that cooking from scratch declined. When microwaves first hit the market in the early 1970s, they were initially seen as a novelty. However, once food manufacturers realized they had an unlimited market for packaged foods that could easily be heated up in only minutes, they increased their offerings and the sales of these foods exploded. The homemade broth and stocks as well as fresh vegetables and whole grains that had once been the basis for so many meals disappeared, to be replaced by packaged and microwavable food laden with chemicals—and soon after that, increasingly created from GMOs.

What Are GMOs?

GMOs are foods produced from organisms that have been manipulated in laboratories by chemicals to change their DNA, or genetic structure. At first this was thought to be a good idea, as the process could add genetic characteristics that would be helpful to farmers and consumers— characteristics such as the ability for fruit to ripen after harvesting, the production of fewer seeds in a lemon, or increased resistance to pesticides

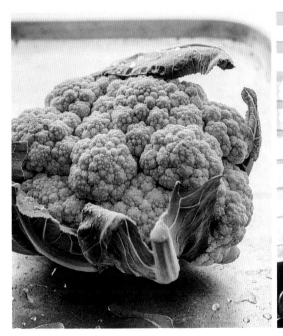
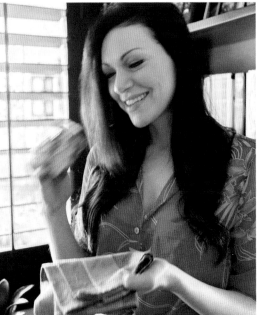

(which makes crops less likely to be damaged by bugs). Farmers often lost entire crops to weeds that choked the fields, and they desperately needed some kind of help to eradicate these issues. What if an herbicide could be created that killed the weeds and not the crops? What if scientists could make genetic changes to the good crops that would make them resistant to the effects of the herbicides on the weeds? That altruistic concept was what led to GMOs being released into the world.

But as millions have found out, GMOs aren't benign. Instead it's like when Bruce Banner gets caught in the blast of gamma radiation and he's cursed to turn into the Hulk in times of stress. GMO-tainted food is literally being Hulk-ified. A perfectly round tomato or fungus-resistant corn might be highly desirable to the food and pesticide industry, but they are highly undesirable to a human body.

Not only is our food being Hulked out, but when your liver attempts to process this fare, it gets super-stressed trying to decipher what exactly this fake food is and how to get rid of it.

The most common crops that have become GMO in the United States are corn, soybeans, canola (used for oil), cotton, cottonseed (used for oil), papaya, alfalfa, and sugar beets. Think about this. GMO food crops are the most prevalent ingredients found in nearly all packaged foods—especially if they contain high-fructose corn syrup, which is made from corn. All animal feed that is not certified to be hormone free is genetically modified. (Animals that aren't fed grass are supplied with corn or soy, which are at the top of the GMO list.)

Clearly, if an animal eats GMO feed, when you eat the meat, you ingest the GMOs, too. In addition, these GMO food crops are found in a huge range of products: packaged bakery goods, cosmetics, power bars (alfalfa is a cheap protein replacement), most oils that aren't organic, *any* kind of fast food, ice creams, jellies, and much more.

There have been extensive studies performed on GMOs and their effects on food. The first patent was issued in 1980, and the first GMO crop—the Flavr Savr tomato, genetically engineered for a longer shelf life—was approved for production in 1992, the same year the FDA claimed that GMOs were "not inherently dangerous" and therefore didn't need strict regulation. Ever since, according to the EPA (Environmental Protection Agency), the USDA (US Department of Agriculture), the NAS (National Academy of Sciences), and the AMA (American Medical Association), GMOs are safe.

Yet here is the enormous problem with that belief. Even these organizations have conceded that no scientifically rigorous long-term double-blind studies (the industry standard) have ever been done on GMOs. Think about the FDA's 1992 declaration. They made it the same year that a GMO tomato was approved! How could they possibly know what GMOs might or might not do over a person's life-span? The GMO foods simply haven't been around long enough. So while scientists can claim that no side effects are "proven"—and that therefore GMOs are safe for all consumption over your entire life-span—that's only because no rigorous studies have been done to prove them.

GMOs are highly regulated for use in the European Union, Australia, and many other countries, and they are banned outright in many areas within those countries. Sixty-four countries, including all those in the European Union, Australia, Russia, and China, mandate the labeling of any food that contains any GMOs. America is making improvements, but not fast enough, and we are seeing a skyrocketing of ills and obesity that is a result of our probing, injecting, and manipulating our food. We as a nation need to support getting our food back to its natural state and out of a lab.

This back-to-basics approach is exactly what we want to achieve with the Stash Plan. Untainted, unprocessed, wholesome food that your body can recognize and utilize for nourishment and vitality—it's not too much to ask, it's not overly difficult, and we're going to show you how it's done.

The Glyphosate Connection

Crucial to the discussion of GMOs and their danger is a chemical called glyphosate. *All* of us have had some contact with glyphosate one way or another throughout our lifetimes—unless you've been living in a mountain village in Tibet, eating only the local, untainted food and nothing else. In which case, you're one of the lucky few!

Glyphosate is found in over 750 different products. It is the key ingredient in herbicides sprayed on our food crops, and has a toxic effect as it is sprayed over crops and is detectable in the air before it seeps into the soil and water sources. Not only can glyphosate cause a range of illnesses, particularly those affecting the blood and kidneys, but it has a devastating effect on the environment, as its use creates super-weeds that are even more herbicide resistant, leading to more chemical use and reduced sustainability.

One of the primary reasons is that GMO crops—predominately soy, corn, and cotton—need to be genetically engineered is so that they remain highly tolerant of pesticides and herbicides. That means that much higher levels of these chemicals contained in pesticides and herbicides are used on crops, as the plants themselves can withstand their use without any damage.

It's a very scary double whammy. Not only are the crops GMO, but they are treated with toxic chemicals in order to kill the weeds that can stunt the crop growth and make harvesting difficult.

The most commonly used herbicide on corn and soy crops is composed predominately of glyphosate as well as another chemical, polyoxyethylene-amine (try saying *that* three times in a row), or POEA, which is a surfactant used to enhance glyphosate's effectiveness. POEA is highly toxic and has been proven to interfere with hormonal levels in many animals, including humans.

In fact, research published in *The Lancet Oncology* in March 2015 that studied the carcinogenicity of several pesticides and herbicides concluded that "glyphosate has been detected in the blood and urine of agricultural workers, indicating absorption. Soil microbes degrade glyphosate to aminomethylphosphonic acid (AMPA). Blood AMPA detection after poisonings suggests intestinal microbial metabolism in humans. Glyphosate and glyphosate formulations induced DNA and chromosomal damage in mammals, and in human and animal cells in vitro." In other words, glyphosates aren't just damaging us—they are damaging future generations as well.

As a result, the Working Group classified glyphosate as "probably carcinogenic to humans." The International Agency for Research on Cancer, a division of the World Health Organization (WHO), therefore classified glyphosate in the category of "probable or possible carcinogens."

One of the biggest issues with glyphosate herbicides is that they are often used to kill weeds right before crops are harvested. This means that consumers can unwittingly get a whopping dose of it from a wide range of foods—even from those you might not expect. It's not just fruits and vegetables that you have to look out for; products that are made from those pesticide-laden foods may also have lots of pesticides, too. So if the corn used to make your cornmeal was tainted with glyphosate, for example, you may be unwittingly at risk for its side effects.

IT'S NOT JUST *fruits and vegetables* **THAT YOU HAVE TO** *look out for.*

There is a simple explanation for glyphosate's dangers. The component that stops the weeds (and other non-GMO plants) from growing does so by inhibiting a specific metabolic pathway, the shikimate pathway, in plants. This pathway is what absorbs the nutrients and the water plants need in order to stay alive. If it's blocked by the chemicals found in herbicides and pesticides, the plant can't grow properly, and it dies.

The shikimate pathway does not exist in people or in animals, which is why companies that use glyphosate in their products have been able to claim that it has no effect on human cells, and therefore it is safe for the human body to ingest glyphosate-tainted foods. But here's the catch: While it is entirely correct that there is no shikimate pathway in human cells, it *does* exist in our intestines. Not in the cells of our intestines. In the trillions of beneficial *bacteria* that live there. In fact, each individual gut bacteria has its own shikimate pathway.

And guess what has an extremely toxic effect on this intestinal bacteria? *Glyphosate.* Whether you eat food contaminated with glyphosate, or when you inhale or absorb any herbicides or pesticides, they cross over the shikimate pathway in your gut flora, causing nutritional deficiencies and toxins in your system. In fact, the glyphosate does to humans and animals what it does to plants—stops nutrients from being absorbed and pokes holes in the walls of each beneficial bacteria. When those holes are created, it causes a chemical reaction within the intestine that turns the good bacteria into a highly toxic substance, making a very unstable environment inside the person, baby, animal, or fetus. This hostile environment can cause many issues including leaky gut, bloating, irritable bowel syndrome, acid reflux, and more.

Not all bacteria are bad for us, like the ones that cause illness. Our intestines are chock-full of enormous quantities of beneficial bacteria, or gut flora, that help us digest our food. We have so many gut bacteria, in fact, that they outnumber our cells *ten to one.* A June 2012 study in the journal *Nutrition in Clinical Practice* showed that microorganisms in the human gastrointestinal tract form an intricate living fabric of natural controls affecting body weight, energy, and nutrition.

What happens when the good bacteria is wiped out? Not only can you feel crummy, but you can end up with a compromised immune system, making it easier for you to become ill with opportunistic infections. We believe this is one of the reasons why the typical standard American diet is so unhealthy, as it can potentially trigger gastrointestinal problems, obesity, diabetes, heart disease, depression, autism, infertility, cancer, and Alzheimer's. How appropriate that the abbreviation for the standard American diet is S.A.D.

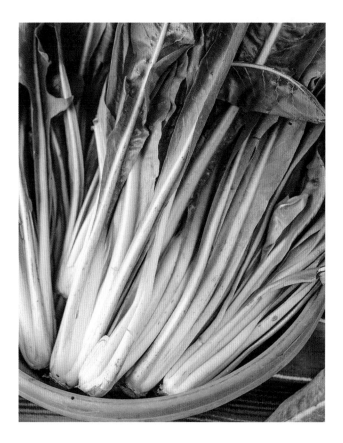

We also believe this is the missing link explaining why gut health is so compromised in so many millions of people, and why so many autoimmune diseases (such as rheumatoid arthritis and celiac disease), diabetes, autism spectrum disorders, depression, and food sensitivities are on the rise. All of them have the common denominator of compromised gut flora in the body. When the colonies of flora are compromised, this allows pathogens to produce toxins and in turn causes inflammation. Much as in *Star Wars*, Luke Skywalker has to use the Force to protect against the dark side; we need to protect our healthy good gut bacteria with the Force (the Stash Plan) so the dark side (evil invaders) don't take it over.

In 2015, we were able to speak at length with Jeffrey Smith, executive director of the Institute for Responsible Technology and the leading consumer advocate promoting healthier non-GMO choices. He explained that thousands of doctors are now prescribing non-GMO diets for themselves and their patients, and he says these doctors are seeing their patients get better from a variety of diseases and disorders.

"I do believe there is a causation that's happening, and I do believe that numerous diseases are being increased and exacerbated because of the use of GMOs and Roundup," Smith said to us. "And I know this because when people get rid of GMOs and Roundup, they get better from the same type of diseases and disorders that are afflicting the land animals fed GMOs and Roundup. Similarly, when livestock get taken off of GMOs, they get better from same type of categories that humans get better from and pets."

The Second Brain = Your Gut

THE WORD *GUT* is tossed around a lot these days. Gut flora, gut health, gut issues—they all refer to your intestinal tract. This includes the stomach, duodenum (the initial segment of the small intestine where nutrients are absorbed), small intestine, and large intestine. Your gut is responsible for digesting food, absorbing nutrients, and expelling waste. All these processes need beneficial gut flora to do their jobs properly.

So imagine the stress our guts go through when we ingest GMO-ridden food and chemicals that kill our gut bacteria. Most of us don't think about how stressed out our organs can become as they try to manage what we put in our bodies; it shouldn't take a heart attack for you to think about the stress on your arteries or the heart muscle itself. Yet a typical American diet is guaranteed to dump a load of stress on your gallbladder, liver, and small intestine, like your boss coming in at four o'clock on a Friday with a new project for you to finish before the weekend. The whole point of the Stash Plan is to leave your gallbladder and liver worry-free and stress-free and therefore fully able to fulfill their natural functions without getting stuck. It's time to pay attention to our all too often neglected intestinal organs and the beneficial flora that live inside them. Pamper 'em and treat 'em right. They're our second brain.

PACKAGED FOODS WITH THE HIGHEST GMO LEVELS

According to the Union of Concerned Scientists, these foods all have high levels of GMOs. Note that their primary ingredients are corn and/or soy.

- Aunt Jemima Pancake Mix
- Ball Park Franks
- Betty Crocker Bac-O's Bacon Flavor Bits
- Boca Burger Chef Max's Favorite
- Duncan Hines Cake Mix
- Enfamil ProSobee Soy Formula
- Frito-Lay Corn Chips
- Gardenburger
- General Mills Total Corn Flakes Cereal
- Heinz 2 Baby Food
- Jiffy Corn Muffin Mix
- Kellogg's Corn Flakes
- MorningStar Farms Better'n Burgers
- Nabisco Snackwell's Granola Bars
- Nestle Carnation Alsoy Infant Formula
- Old El Paso Taco Shells
- Ovaltine Malt Powdered Beverage Mix
- Post Blueberry Morning Cereal
- Quaker Chewy Granola Bars
- Quaker Yellow Corn Meal
- Similac Isomil Soy Formula
- Ultra Slim Fast

As you know, the neurons, or nerve cells, in our brains fire electrical impulses so our thoughts can be processed and our bodies can function. Humans have about 100 billion brain neurons, and each one communicates in its own unique way to transmit necessary information to our muscles, glands, and organs. What you likely don't know is that our gut flora have *twice as many* neurons as the brain, as well as its own separate communication processes within itself. In addition, research by the UCLA Division of Digestive Diseases published in 2013 showed that gut flora directly communicates with the brain: "Intestinal flora has protective metabolic and immune function and is able to 'cross talk' with the nervous system."

OUR GUT FLORA HAVE *twice as many* NEURONS AS THE BRAIN.

Perhaps we shouldn't think of our gut as the second brain but as an equal to the brain in our skulls. After all, both the central nervous system and the nervous system in the gastrointestinal tract are created by identical tissue in a developing fetus. And like the brain inside our skull, the brain inside our abdomen fires off hundreds of thousands of sensory outputs within itself and the rest of our bodies.

Think about the effect GMOs and toxic chemicals like glyphosate have on our gut bacteria. If the liver can't do its job as our chemical filtration system, these evil invaders pass into the duodenum. They attack our gut bacteria, just like they do to bugs and weeds, stopping the shikimate pathway and killing them.

Another important factor about our gut bacteria is that neurons in our gut produce neurotransmitters just like the brain does (but double as many). One of these neurotransmitters is serotonin, which correlates with your mood, mental health, anxiety, excitement, anger, depression, and mental clarity. Funny how a depressed person is often prescribed antidepressants to raise brain serotonin levels—without considering that addressing the gut levels of serotonin might be a much healthier and speedier way to tackle the problem. Changing your diet to the Stash Plan can increase your positive emotions, increase your energy levels, and sharpen your mental focus—and of course the weight naturally comes off.

Why does the Stash Plan repair and feed your gut? One of the most potent reasons is broth. It's essential for gut repair, and nourishing broth will help micronutrients be properly absorbed in your small intestine, even if your gut is damaged when you start the program. Broth replenishes the enzymes, bone marrow, and minerals that have been depleted from your diet for many years. The Stash Plan food is filled with active cultures to help rebuild and strengthen your gut flora—creating a new foundation of health to move forward.

Because GMOs, herbicides, and pesticides have such a potent effect on gut bacteria, it's very important to understand more about digestion—especially as gut problems have a direct impact on why we can be so tired, depressed, and overweight.

What Happens When You Eat: The Link from the Gut to the Gallbladder and Liver

Let's look at the journey of a piece of food from the moment you decide to eat it:

- Food goes into your mouth.

- **As you chew,** your teeth grind the food into smaller pieces, and enzymes in your saliva immediately start to break it down.

- The food particles travel down your esophagus into your stomach.

- **The stomach's job,** along with why we chew our food in the first place, is solely to break down food so that the small intestine can then absorb the nutrients. Last time we checked, our stomachs didn't have bicuspids, molars, or eyeteeth!

  Many people erroneously believe that nutrients are absorbed through your stomach. Instead, the stomach's function is to use its acids, along with the bile from your liver, to process the food you've eaten into a sort of mush that is emulsified enough into a semifluid state so it can then be small and soft enough to be able to pass through the duodenum into your small intestine. (Remember, the amount of bile released depends on how much fat is contained in whatever you've just eaten.) The technical term for this emulsion is *chyme,* which is derived from the Greek word for juice.

ELIZABETH

From 2005 to 2010 I would marvel with my clients, "Where did all of our health go?" I began to see more and more autoimmune issues; clients were suddenly coming in with multiple sclerosis, fibromyalgia, lupus, psoriasis, and juvenile arthritis. The children I saw invariably had low muscle tone and were easily fatigued, and had delayed motor development, excessive sleepiness, and irritability. The health implications in gut bacteria acquired from birth determines the profound dynamic interaction between your gut, your brain, and your immune system. Research done by Dr. Natasha Campbell-McBride, published in May 2014, concluded that the majority of people she studied had poor gut health due to poor diet and toxic exposures. She also showed that good gut health is particularly crucial for pregnant woman and young children. Campbell-McBride proposes a nutritional program she calls GAPS (which stands for Gut and Psychology Syndrome) to promote a healthy interaction between the gut, the brain, and the immune system. For me, the *most* amazing part of the GAPS diet is that drinking homemade and organic meat or fish broth is an essential part of your breakfast. This way, it's the first food to hit your empty stomach in the morning, and it will heal the gut lining without the interference of other food.

The issues my clients had were usually autoimmune disorders, as well as infertility, depression, and food allergies. Early in my practice, I had started to theorize that if my clients with these health conditions changed their diet to what has since become the Stash Plan, and if they came to class two to three times a week for targeted stretching, their bodies would respond by repairing, strengthening, and energizing to ignite self-created healing. It worked! All of my clients with these issues had advanced symptoms, but they were thrilled and astonished when they soon felt relief.

Another reason that GMO crops can wreak havoc on our bodies is that they just don't contain the same essential nutrients as their non-GMO counterparts. Dr. Donald Huber of the UK-based Institute of Science in Society, a think tank designed to provide unbiased information for the public good, is an expert in the toxicity of genetically engineered foods. His studies have proven that GMO crops are depleted of up to 95 percent of essential minerals, such as calcium, magnesium, copper, iron, and zinc.

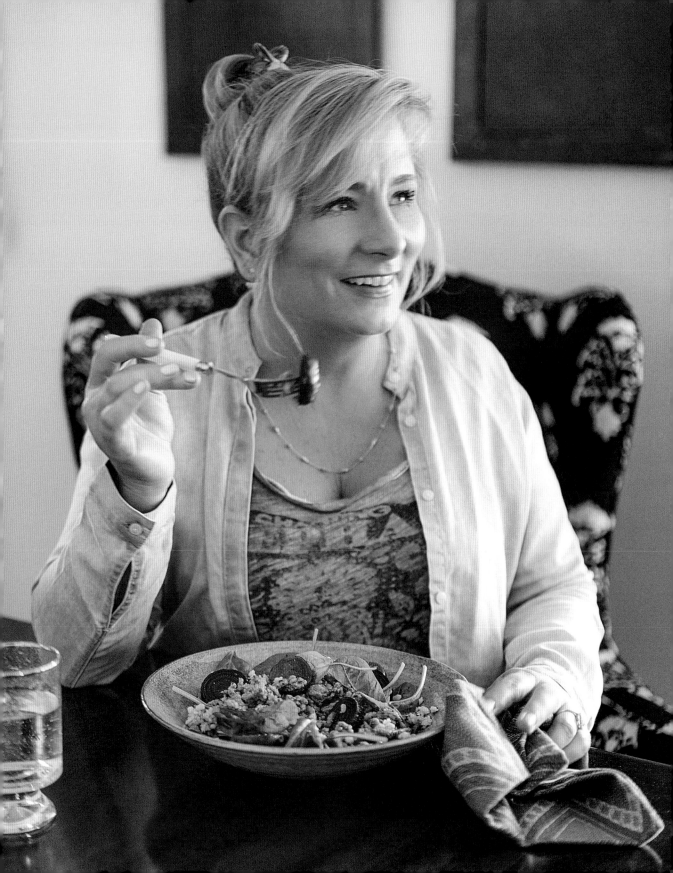

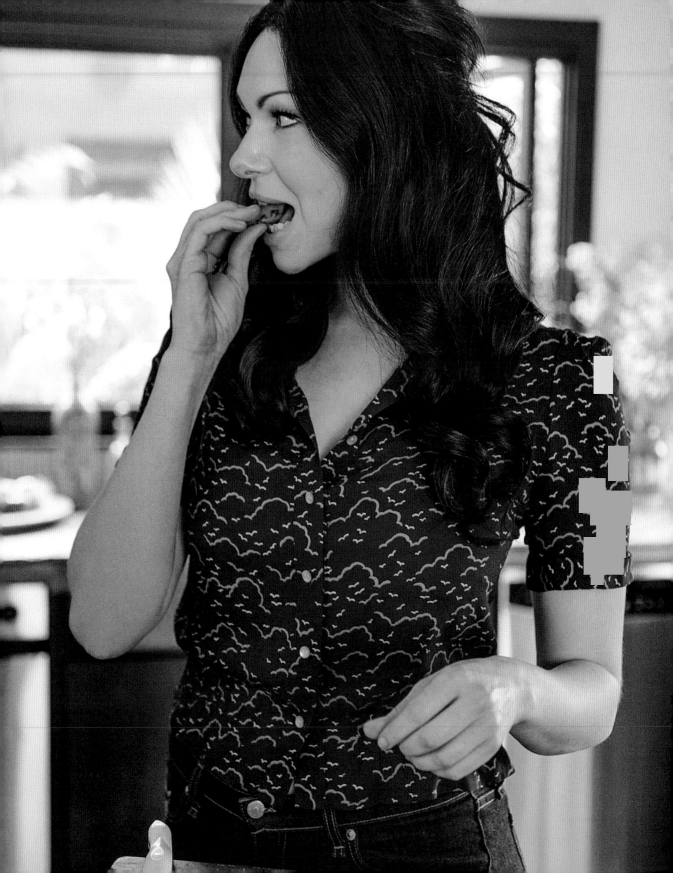

- **After your food is pulverized into chyme,** it moves along to the duodenum. This is where the stars of the Stash Plan—our superheroes, the gallbladder and liver—kick into high gear. The liver calls on the gallbladder for more bile to further break down your food so that its nutrients can be absorbed properly. From here, it continues into the small intestine for further nutrient absorption. The small intestine's job is basically to selectively absorb what nutrients are needed and good for us, and reject what is bad. Good nutrients are passed through the intestinal walls into the bloodstream, where they are carried along to various cells so they can function. This process is aided by the teeming colonies of bacteria in your gut.

- **Next stop is the large intestine.** There, bacterial fermentation converts the chyme into fecal matter; during this process, B vitamins and vitamin K are released, along with the gas we all know so well. The chyme moves along thanks to peristalsis, which is the propulsive action of the intestinal muscles. (As when a pastry chef decorates a cake, the hand that squeezes the pastry bag pushes the icing out of the tip, providing this propulsion/peristalsis action.) As this is happening, water is constantly being absorbed by the large intestine in order to solidify and condense the fecal matter into pieces firm enough to expel through your rectum and out your anus.

  If, however, you eat junk, fake, or GMO-tainted food, this entire cycle goes awry. This is what happens instead:

- **Your liver tries to decipher** what has just been ingested. As with normal real food, after you take a bite and start to chew, enzymes start to digest and pulverize the food in your mouth, and it then goes down your esophagus and into your stomach.

LAURA

• • • • •

I think all of us have had an experience with heartburn—that awful burning in your chest and your throat—at some point. One of the main reasons you get heartburn is due to what we just touched on: the food your body can't figure out, and the constant need for more bile to break it down. All of this bile equals heartburn. I always think it's funny when I see ads on TV for heartburn aids that just cover up the problem, when the solution is to change what you're eating in the first place. Food on the Stash Plan will never have you at your local drugstore reaching for Tums or Zantac.

- **Here is where the problems start.** The liver is trying to decipher what has just come down the pipe, but is stumped. Flustered, the liver calls to the gallbladder for more bile, which is needed to break down these unrecognizable foods. The food stops getting digested properly and isn't churned into chyme. At a certain point, the liver gives up and passes the buck. This partially digested food is passed along to the duodenum.

- **Once the food is in the duodenum,** the liver decides to try again but still can't decipher what this stuff is, so it sends more urgent signals to the gallbladder for even more bile to help break the food down. (Think of it as begging for more ammo against the evil invaders.) But this just doesn't work, because it can't. Your body just can't perceive this food as *real*. Your body wants it *out*, so it's moved along to the small intestine. At this point, of course, many nutrients have not been absorbed yet through the walls of the duodenum, because they could not be recognized as safe. Nor are they recognized as safe farther along in the small intestine.

  In addition, when the bile gets backed up and undigested food moves along slowly, the villi—fingerlike projections that protrude from the lining of the intestinal wall, akin to the tentacle-looking sponges that move over a car in an automated car wash— flatten out and get stuck to the side of the intestines. As villi absorb nutrients into the blood, their flattening also impedes the absorption of nutrients.

- **This renegade mixture** keeps moving along toward the large intestine so it can be expelled as waste. Here, however, it slows down even further and gets sluggish because it hasn't been churned into chyme and is still only partially digested. The large intestine wants to get rid of it but can't, so it keeps pulling water from the fecal matter, causing it to become hard and stuck—you know this as constipation. This waste material then sits in your large intestine, rotting and fermenting, giving us gas, and backing things up.

- **Leaky gut syndrome might also ensue.** This is a condition that has finally made it into mainstream medical discussions after being dismissed as wholly impossible by many doctors over the years. Also called increased intestinal permeability, leaky gut syndrome is a condition that can arise

CONSTIPATION IS A REAL PROBLEM

Constipation isn't just an annoyance. It can lead to serious problems.

Every body has a different poop schedule that is normal for them. Those who eat an extremely healthy diet full of fiber poop after every meal if they don't have a systemic problem. Our bodies are designed to get rid of waste three times a day. When you're constipated, however, you can go for days (or longer in severe cases) without pooping, and this wreaks havoc on your entire digestive system.

Constipation can be caused by processed food; GMO food; a diet lacking in fiber, vegetables, and fruit, especially if it is heavy in simple carbohydrates such as sugar and white flour; emotional distress; certain prescription medications; air pollutants; and a lack of regular exercise.

The reason? Our bodies are continually absorbing water from the food we eat at a constant rate through the walls of the large intestine. If, however, the stool isn't moving through the intestine fast enough due to slowed-down peristalsis, the gut responds by pulling too much water away from the waste matter and through its walls. The newly forming stools can then become dry and hard, sometimes almost like tar. This dried-up stool makes it much harder to poop normally.

Constipation doesn't make much sense to the average person. It's caused by their large intestines absorbing too *much* water—but constipation sufferers are told to drink *more* water to get things moving again.

What helps alleviate constipation is, yes, a lot more water, and more fiber in the diet, which will add bulk to the stool and help soften it. Pure unsweetened organic aloe vera juice also helps. Elizabeth tells the parents of constipated babies to get them off soy formula, to make their own organic pureed baby food, and to practice baby abdominal massage. She has had the same results with older children, especially when they eliminate packaged foods from their diet. These include any packaged foods made with high-fructose corn syrup, artificial colorings, nonorganic peanut butter and jelly, frozen pizza, fast food, dried noodles like ramen, packaged meals like Lunchables and mac and cheese, deli meats, Wonder Bread, and nonorganic chips and snacks. Those who tend to get constipated are very pleased when they go on the Stash Plan, as one of its immediate benefits is smooth and easy elimination.

when the lining of the intestine is damaged, making it less able to protect the internal environment as well as filter needed nutrients and other substances in the body. When this happens, bacteria and their toxins, incompletely digested proteins and fats, and waste meant to be excreted (not absorbed) can "leak" out of the intestines into the bloodstream.

If these molecules, now merrily floating along in your blood, react with your body's immune system—especially if they are similar to pre-existing tissue—this can trigger an autoimmune reaction, leading to gastrointestinal problems such as bloating, excessive gas and cramps, fatigue, food sensitivities, joint pain, and rashes.

Elizabeth's Theory
ON THE LIVER AND HUNGER

SO MANY OF MY CLIENTS, like Laura, are hungry no matter what they do! They've tried eating six small meals a day; high-protein diets; all-liquid diets; no-carb or no-gluten diets—you name it. My hunch was that this constant hunger was due to the relationship between the liver and the brain.

The part of the brain that regulates hunger is the hypothalamus. Interestingly enough, the hypothalamus is divided into two sections—the lateral and the paraventricular. The lateral section deals with habit—what you have always eaten throughout your life or what you're familiar with. The paraventricular section deals with cravings; you may feel hungry and you want a specific food, almost as if your body is telling you *exactly* what it needs and making you want to do anything to get it.

Now, when we eat, most of our food is converted into glucose, or blood sugar, during digestion. The liver transforms glucose into fat for storage, so it can be used when needed. When our glucose levels are low, the liver sends a strong signal to the lateral hypothalamus—its habit section—for food that will quickly give us energy. With the Stash Plan, you'll already have your fridge full of amazing food that will nourish your gallbladder and liver, providing maximum nutrition.

You'll also become much more in tune with your body and what it truly needs. This directly affects your paraventricular hypothalamus—the cravings part. You'll soon find yourself reaching for exactly what your body needs from the stashes you've already prepared. A fully nourished body is one that diminishes your hunger and helps you get rid of bad habits and harmful cravings, replacing them instead with a desire for food that is always going to be good for you. You're going to walk away from those bad foods like you're forgetting about an old flame that wasn't the best relationship . . . to meeting a hot new one with energy and a lust for life! You'll look back and say, "What was I thinking?" We understand, because sometimes it's hard to realize exactly what's going on while you're *in* it. But, now with the Stash Plan foods, it's like being with someone who makes you feel good, who nourishes your mind and body, and gives you the energy that makes you feel like you can do anything. That will help you lose weight, get healthier, and look amazing . . . sign us up!

The other part of hunger is lack of nutrients. This is a legitimate constant hunger—because your body is starved of the nutrients it needs. So you eat some more. But if you eat the same kind of fake GMO-laden foods, the same cycle starts all over again.

When you eat GMOs, you're both eating more and *storing* more. Why? Because GMOs trigger your body to go into starvation mode because you're not absorbing nutrients. When this happens and you're not getting the nutrients your body requires, your metabolism slows down because it believes you're starving, clicking back into that evolutionary drive to conserve energy as much as possible in times of famine. This is also why starvation diets don't work. Cave dwellers never knew where their next meal was coming from, so their bodies evolved to store fat easily when nourishment was not readily available. Now, when we can eat whatever and whenever we want and don't have to hunt for our food with a club and rocks, we still have cave-dweller-type metabolisms primed to hold on to fat when we're starving. Following the Stash Plan will put an end to this cycle.

> A FULLY *nourished body* IS ONE THAT *diminishes your hunger* AND HELPS YOU GET RID OF *bad habits* AND HARMFUL *cravings*.

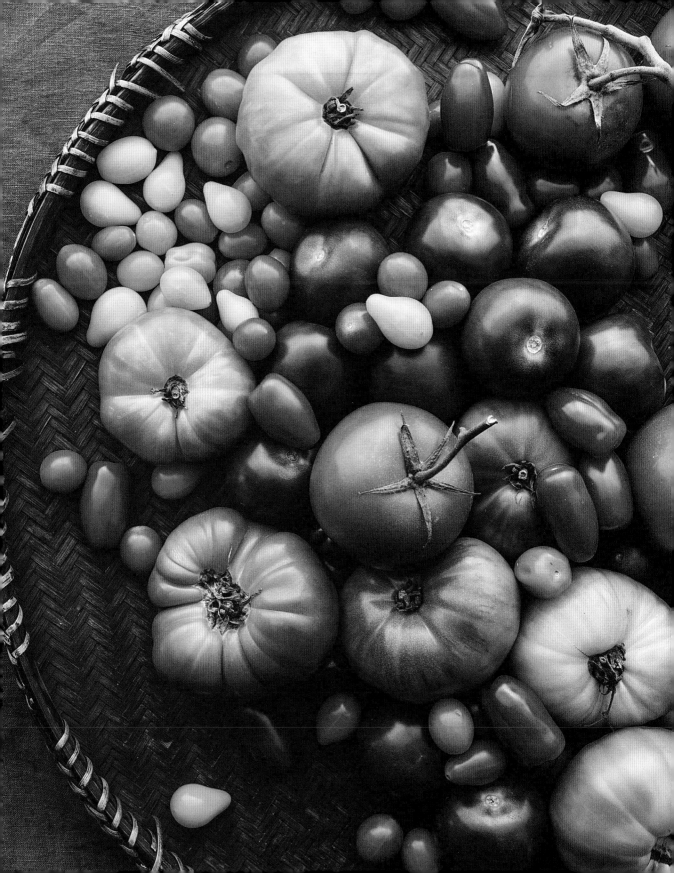

UNDERSTANDING
the Lymphatic System

OUR LYMPHATIC SYSTEM is our internal immune system. We have twice as much lymphatic fluid in our body as blood, as well as twice as many lymph vessels as blood vessels. It's not an overstatement to say that keeping your lymph system in order can improve your health and maybe even save your life—yet few Americans understand what lymph is or how and why it works.

In fact, an estimated 10 million Americans have some form of lymphedema, or swelling of tissue/swollen lymph nodes, which is caused by a problematic lymphatic system. They often think this bloating is water weight or fat, when it's not. Elizabeth noticed this, in particular, with approximately 80 percent of her clients of all ages starting about a decade ago, and it has progressively gotten worse. Before that, it was very rare. Something has been triggering all this sluggish lymph—which turns into bloat!

The four parts of the lymphatic system are the lymph itself, the lymph nodes, the lymph vessels, and lymphatic fluid that flows freely through your body. The name comes from the Latin word *lympha,* which means water. You've seen lymph if you get a superficial cut and a clear fluid seeps out before the blood does; lymph carries useful components such as white blood cells (infection fighters), fats, and hormones to the places they're needed. Of course we know that fats are what the bile breaks down, and we know hormones are produced and regulated in the liver. Thus the harmony of the lymph, liver, and gallbladder is crucial.

We discussed the lymphatic system in Chapter 3, when we explained how the lymph also acts as a waste disposal system, collecting toxins, viruses, dead and diseased cells, and cancerous cells that need to pass through the lymph nodes for filtration.

The lymph nodes are the second part of the system. They're mainly clustered like grapes in areas such as the neck, elbow, armpit, groin, back of the head, and the back of the legs. When the nodes become swollen, it means there is an infection or blockage somewhere in the lymphatic

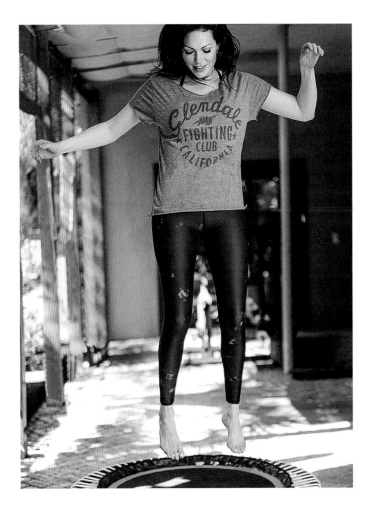

system. As a major component of the immune system, the lymph, lymph white blood cells (lymphocytes), and antibodies defend your body from infection and foreign invaders. When you think about where nodes are clustered in the body, it's not surprising that certain cancers like breast and prostate are on the rise. If there are nodes clustered under the arm-pit, when these nodes become full, naturally these pathogens and invaders will go to the closest part of the body—namely, your breast. The same thing happens with the nodes around the prostate. Think about other areas where this could be happening as well.

HELP YOUR LYMPH FLOW MORE SMOOTHLY

As you know, your heart is responsible for pumping blood in your circulatory system. The lymphatic system doesn't have its own pump, so it can easily be stagnant—it works primarily by being squeezed by your muscles. Here's how to help your lymph to flow smoothly:

- Drink at least sixty-four ounces of filtered water every day.

- Do at least twenty minutes of a rebounding type of exercise. You can do this by bouncing on an individual trampoline or rebounder, jumping rope, or skipping. These exercises pump this fluid because the muscles squeeze lymph during these activities, moving it through.

- Do deep abdominal breathing exercises. This allows the lymph to flow smoothly. This type of exercise is ideal for older people who aren't able to do strenuous activity.

- Try dry skin brushing. The lymph naturally moves in the direction toward the heart, so brushing upward on the legs, torso, and arms in that direction will help the lymphatic flow. Use a soft dry brush with natural bristles; these can be found in any health or wellness store.

- Using an infrared sauna a few times a week helps and supports the Stash Plan by keeping your toxins moving through and calming your central nervous system, among many other positive effects!

  Infrared saunas are very different from traditional saunas. Infrared waves penetrate the thickest part of any solid object. In the human body, that happens to be the liver. When the wave hits the liver, it vibrates deep into it and pulls out old toxins and also kills off viruses and bacteria. Traditional saunas simply pull water from your body.

- Follow the Stash Plan. Our food plan avoids saturated fats, sugars, and refined or processed foods, which will greatly improve your lymphatic circulation.

The third and fourth part of the lymphatic system are the lymph vessels (which unlike blood vessels, only carry fluid away from the tissues) and the free flowing lymphatic fluid in the nooks and crannies of your body.

This is how your lymphatic system reacts when you eat something your body doesn't recognize, like a Hostess Ding Dong. The Ding Dong goes to the stomach, where the liver doesn't know what to do with it, and then this undigested renegade food is passed along to the duodenum. It still can't be deciphered and is passed through the intestines and out of your body. Now, as you know, the large intestine's job is to pull water from fecal matter and propel the feces toward the exit. But if the water that is being pulled out is full of evil invaders—thanks to whatever you ate or drank or smoked—the lymph rushes to deal with it and remove these impostors.

If, however, there are too many toxins moving through the large intestine, peristalsis slows down and the gunk in there can become more destructive. Just as your gallbladder and liver can be overwhelmed with the evil invaders, so too can the lymphatic system be overtaken. When that happens, lymph nodes overflow, and the only place for these intruders to go is into the blood. The liver, being your blood's washing machine, now has to try to deal with these guys *again*. It's a constant cycle of "What do we do with this stuff?" Fortunately, the Stash Plan helps you break this cycle.

WHAT CAN YOU DO
about GMOs?

JEFFREY SMITH, a leading consumer advocate promoting healthier non-GMO choices, explains that the way to rid the nation of GMOs "has nothing to do with government policy because that's the power source for Monsanto [the largest producer of Roundup]. Where it lies is in market solutions." Industries and companies must be brought to realize that using GMOs will actually cost them *more* money than *not* using them. This is called pushing that industry or company to the "tipping point." Consumer rejection is a powerful way to create a positive change to a negative action.

In the natural product industry, the tipping point came in March 2013, when the president of Whole Foods realized when a product becomes verified as non-GMO, this increases its sales 15 to 30 percent. In January 2014 Cheerios announced it was non-GMO; then two and a half weeks later Grape-Nuts, Smart Balance, I Can't Believe It's Not Butter, Ben & Jerry's, Hershey, and Chipotle followed suit. Mainstream supermarkets that have brand names everyone knows are now declaring many of their products to be non-GMO.

A survey from the Hartman Group, a consumer research organization, stated that in 2007, 15 percent of Americans were already avoiding and reducing GMOs. In 2014, it was 40 percent—an indication that this issue is highly popular. Corporate ears are perking up in a big way, and corporate leaders are starting to listen now that consumer rejection of these invisible poisons is hurting company profits.

The Center for Food Safety has done an excellent job of highlighting the potential risks of GMOs on human health, including toxicity, allergic reactions, antibiotic resistance, immune suppression, cancer, and loss of nutrition. As they point out: "The FDA also does not require *any* premarket safety testing for GE/GMO foods."

Fortunately, more and more states are requiring GMO labeling and consumers are becoming more aware of their dangers. The goal is to reverse and eliminate systemic illnesses and conditions like chronic gut problems, autistic spectrum disorders, cancer, heart disease, diabetes, and malaise and exhaustion through a systematic eating plan that heals the body. It can be done. There is a light at the end of the tunnel, so you should take heart, because there are solutions to GMO foods and the rampant overuse of pesticides and herbicides like glyphosate:

- **Follow the Stash Plan,** because it will set you on the road to wellness while healing your gallbladder and liver and improving all aspects of the digestive process. The eating plan in this book is vital to your health— and your weight!

- **Eat organic food that is not tainted by GMOs.** The more people buy organic, the lower the prices will become.

- **Demand that all food that is GMO be labeled as such.** Sales of GMO-labeled and third-party-verified as organic items are growing exponentially; according to Whole Foods, in 2012 they were the fastest growing subset of food. Contact your elected representatives, because legislation is being introduced in some states to improve labeling, and this is directly due to public pressure.

- **Avoid using any glyphosate-based herbicides** on your lawn or garden.

- **Educate yourself** about the hazards of GMOs, pesticides, and herbicides, and lobby for better consumer protections from their toxic effects. There are excellent resources online. For example, the Non-GMO Project is a nonprofit organization helping educate and motivate consumers to get involved in the movement (www.nongmoproject.org). Their non-GMO shopping guide is part of the Institute for Responsible Technology, and they've created a downloadable app so you'll always have updated lists handy to advise you on how to shop for non-GMO foods (www.nongmoshoppingguide.com).

- **Many other grassroots organizations** are being formed to help educate people about the dangers of GMOs and the toxins being sprayed on them. Among them are Right to Know GMO, The Future of Food, Food & Water Watch, Just Label It, and the Organic Consumers Association.

- **Make your voice heard.** Food manufacturers listen to their customers, and sometimes they can respond in the most positive of ways. Speak to your health-care providers, too. Print out useful information from some of the sites listed above, and hand it to your doctor. The more that health-care providers know about GMOs, the more likely they are to advise their patients to be on a non-GMO diet.

- **Use the media.** In 1994, for example, countries in the European Union as well as Japan passed laws for approval of GMOs. A research scientist who was involved in the development of GMOs realized soon after these laws were passed that he was wrong, and that GMOs were devastating to human life and the environment. He decided to leak information to a reporter, and within six months, over seven hundred articles appeared throughout Europe and Asia and various countries' governments took action to label and reevaluate the effects of genetically modified foods. American media has not been as responsive, but you can easily call health reporters or bloggers—and speak to the health-conscious shoppers who are already buying $30 million of organic food in this country every year. Do your homework and ask for stories to be written. The more these issues get into the media, the more people can become informed—and the more we can demand that GMOs be removed from our food supply.

- Support advocates like **Sally Fallon of the Weston A. Price Foundation** and bestselling author of *Nourishing Traditions* and *Nourishing Broth*. We spoke to her about the importance of community involvement. Sally stressed the importance of raising awareness and education standards for the health-impeding challenges involving the agricultural industry. These first steps in activism and education are key to achieving food freedom and resolving systemic health issues nationwide. In addition, Jeffrey Smith has a Five-Year Master Plan, which entails raising $5 million dollars each year for five years for educating the public on the use of GMOs and their effects on living things.

- **Encourage GMO labeling nationally.** The goal is to get all GMOs out of American food supply in three years and GMOs out of animal feed within five years.

- **Mommy bloggers are also a vital media force.** Mothers want their children to be safe and healthy. Send them ideas for stories. They have a terrific potential for going viral—and putting and end to GMOs.

LAURA

In all of the books I have read over the years looking for answers to my ailments and weight issues, the information we just covered (I know, it's a lot!) is vital data I had been missing all this time. This chapter actually took us the longest to write because there is so much amazing information we wanted to share with you without overwhelming you. You now have the understanding of what happens in your body when GMOs enter the picture, why we're bloated because of our overtaxed lymphatic system, and how our "second brain" is a vital piece of the feeling good/looking your best/optimizing your health puzzle!

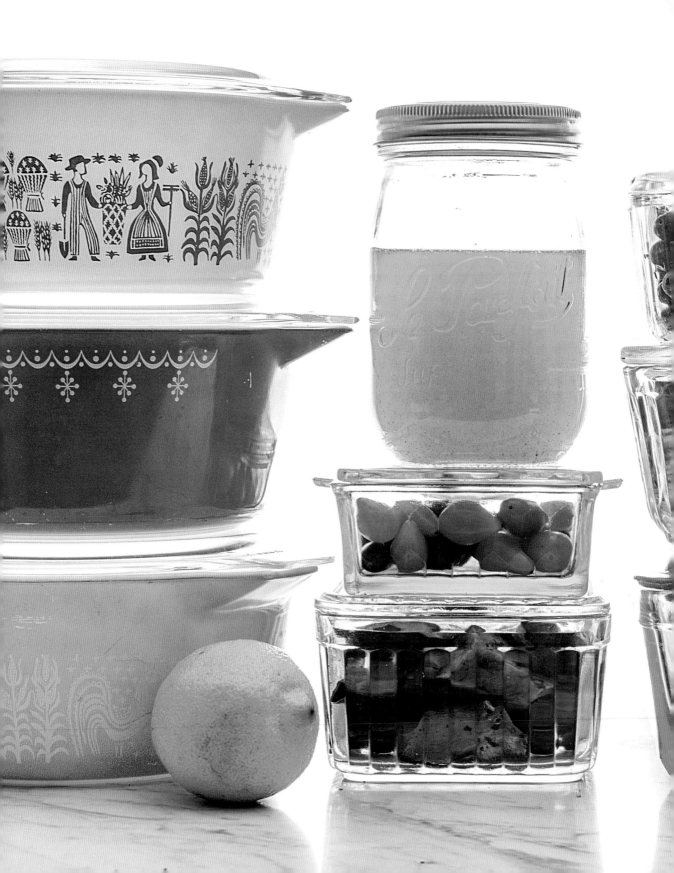

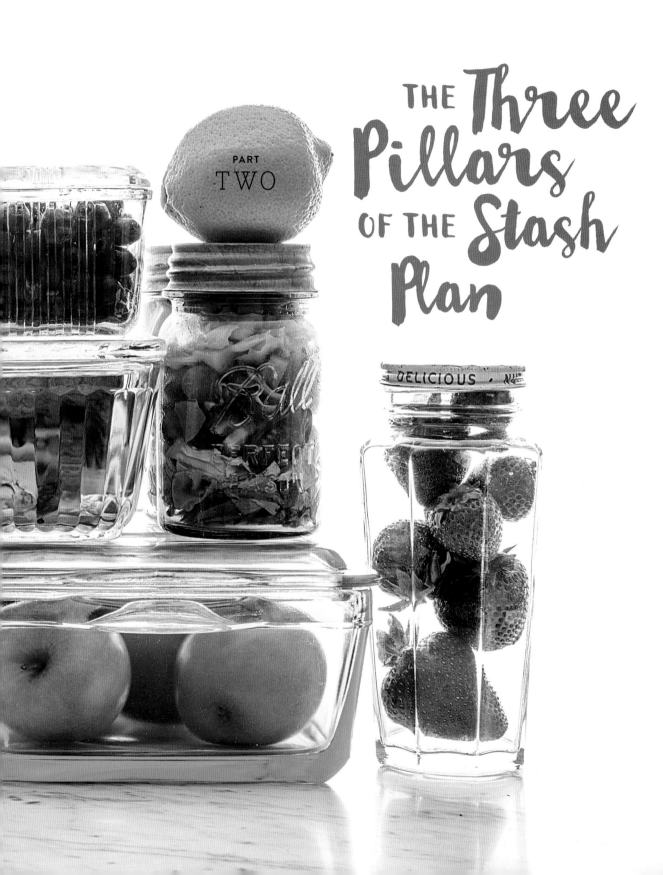

THE *Three* *Pillars* OF THE *Stash* *Plan*

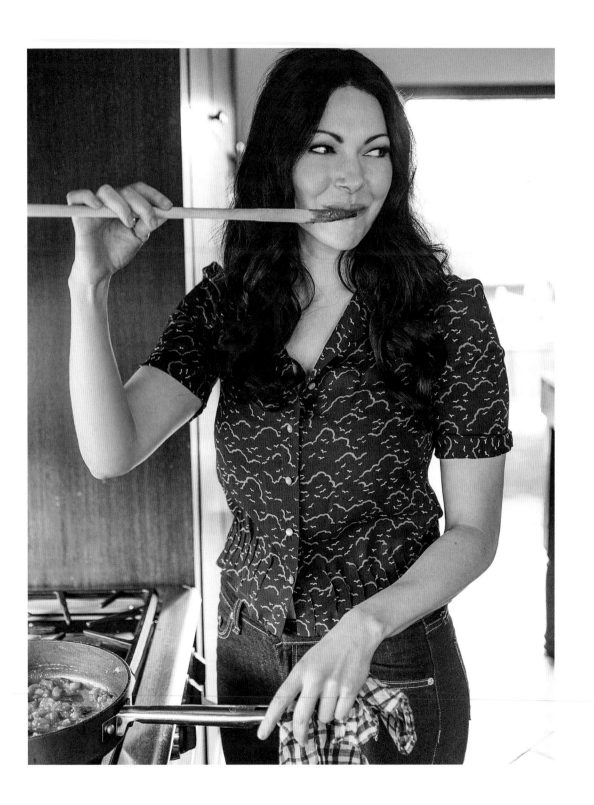

IN THIS PART OF THE BOOK,

you'll learn about the three *dynamic pillars* of the Stash Plan. Think you know why chicken soup makes you feel so good and helps get rid of your colds? *Chapter 5* will give you a primer on the near-magical qualities of broth, and show you how making your own will kick-start your eating plan. In *Chapter 6*, we'll teach you about *antioxidants*—often one of those buzzwords that people tend to throw around without understanding what it means!—as well as the importance of good fats, good *fiber*, and good things to drink. Then in *Chapter 7*, Elizabeth will explain the fundamentals of her marvelous *Muscle Meridian Method*. These are targeted resistance stretches unlike any you've done before.

The POWER OF BROTH

chapter 5

Everyone is familiar with the old wives' tale about the power of chicken soup to help with cold and flu symptoms. It's not just due to the fact that hot liquids are good for you—it's because chicken soup is chicken broth, *made when the bones of the full chicken and vegetables are boiled down for hours to extract maximum micronutrients.*

Whenever you make broth, the boiling process extracts these micronutrients from beef bones (which we like the most for their power-packed micronutrients), whole chickens, whole fish, or vegetables, creating a super-drink with all its nutrients in their most bioavailable form—meaning that they are easily assimilated. The body can very easily drink them up right away, to help heal and strengthen your brain, muscles, joints, and bones from within as well as give your skin a youthful, vibrant glow. Whether you're an athlete healing from an injury, a mom worried about her children's digestive issues, a person wanting optimal health and mental focus, or just someone wanting to restore the radiance of your skin, broth is right for you.

The nutritional punch of these broths makes them one of the most important components of the Stash Plan. The recipes you'll find in Chapter 10 can also be used for flavoring as well as in sauces and dips. We try to cook with them whenever we can to utilize these powerhouse nutrients. You'll never want to use a cube or can of fake broth again. As soon as you start sipping your broths every day, they'll become your new bestie; or better yet, a new significant other who cuddles you, warms you, nourishes your body and soul, and looks *hot* on your arm. Yes, please!

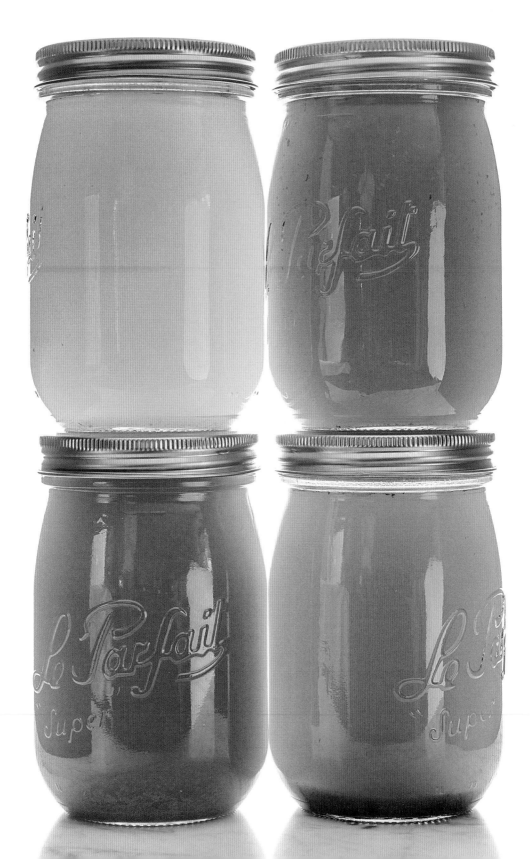

Broth Is the
NEW JUICE

AS YOU KNOW ALREADY, a typical modern diet is overloaded with chemical additives like MSG, sugar, preservatives, trans fats, and runoff from harmful farming practices. What our bodies truly need are the micronutrients found in real, unprocessed food to help heal digestive issues, strengthen immunity, and improve our cardiovascular circulation as well as the movement of cerebral spinal fluid. This is a clear body fluid that moves blood up the spine into the brain (which helps with mood and depression); it also serves as a cushion for the brain and protects it immunologically.

Humans have been drinking broths since our earliest days on earth. Stone soups came first, as the stones were boiled in water to extract their mineral content. As prehistoric men and women became better hunters, they started using marrowbones from the animals they killed to make their broth. Eating this marrow helped these cave dwellers evolve into modern man and woman—by making their bodies and brains stronger and healthier, and with a more powerful immune system allowing them to live longer.

Ancient Greeks and Romans often wrote about the virtues of broth and marrow, particularly when describing how soldiers ate their marrow right before heading out to conquer the enemy. Centuries later, England's Queen Victoria ate marrow on buttered toast every day at teatime, even though it was considered unladylike. She was the queen, however, so all hail . . . well, the *broth* in our case!

Almost every culture throughout history has had broth as a foundation of their diet. In countries where broth is regularly consumed (often on a daily basis), people tend to be less prone to the same health issues that plague those who follow a typical American diet.

For example, in the traditional Japanese and Korean diets, the broth of the ramen soup is by far the most important component. Every spoonful or slurp is savored, and it is considered disrespectful to the chef if even a drop is left at the bottom of the bowl. Ramen chefs take decades to perfect their broth and guard their recipes zealously. Not surprisingly, the heart disease rate in Japan is a third of the American rate.

In the countries of the former Soviet Union, one of their staple foods, beef borsch, is often eaten several times a week, even for breakfast. It is a powerful way to start the day, as beets are great for the creation of new red blood cells, and the beef bones promote deep healing. In Georgia, Uzbekistan, and Tajikistan, cancer death rates are less than half of those in America.

And in China, there are many variations of fish broths. Some are made solely from shellfish, which is great for cartilage. Others use the whole fish, which is a terrific source of omega fatty acids as well as the iodine needed for thyroid regulation (which helps burn fat). The Chinese have far lower levels of rheumatoid arthritis and fibromyalgia than Americans do.

In this country, however, we've shifted away from the traditions of broth making, thinking of broth as something you pour from a can rather than simmer on a stovetop. But if you look at the label of a typical can or box of broth, how many chemicals or artificial flavors have been added to it? How much salt or MSG? How many ingredients can you actually pronounce?

Packaged broth isn't real broth. It might be convenient, but it isn't healing. The Stash Plan broth will give you a new vitality that you may have been missing. It's like feeding your blood—and that in turn feeds the rest of your organs. Some people drink coffee to wake up, have a glass of wine to relax, and keep a pitcher of water on hand for hydration. Drinking bone broth gives you so much more—it's a vital life force. Don't wait until you get a bad cold to think about a steaming bowl of chicken soup. When broth becomes part of your life, you won't get sick as often because you will proactively be building up your immune system.

That's because drinking bone broth is like drinking from the fountain of youth. The nourishing micronutrients go directly into your bloodstream to start healing you immediately. It's rich in cartilage for your joints and bones and builds healthy bone marrow, lowering your risk of a compromised immune system. Bone broth also creates and builds collagen, the protein fibers of our skin responsible for making us look young and vibrant.

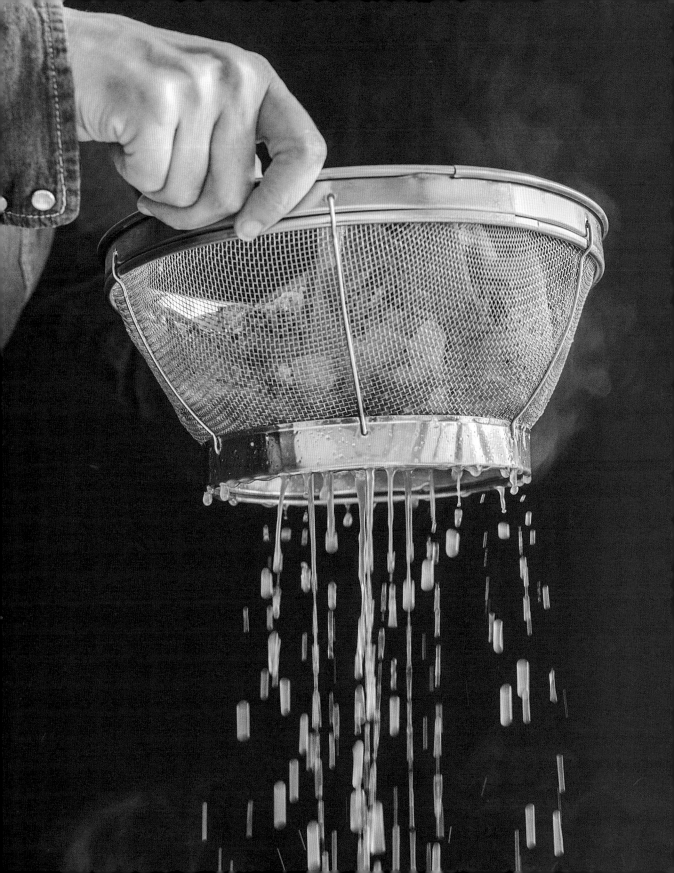

As we age, our collagen levels go from plum to prune. Drinking this amazing tonic helps to slow down this impending fate by restoring healthy collagen levels.

In her bestselling book *Nourishing Broth*, author and nutritionist Sally Fallon explains the principle of "like feeds like," meaning that "broth can give our bones strength and flexibility, our joints cushion and resilience, and our skin a youthful plumpness." This means that if you want healthy collagen, strong bones and cartilage, and clean, healthy bone marrow, eat foods with healthy collagen, strong bones and cartilage, and clean, healthy marrow. In other words, *broth!*

She further explains, "The abundance of collagen in all types of bone broth supports heart health through strong and supple arteries, our vision with healthy corneas, digestion through gut healing, and overall disease prevention via immune system modulation. Broth even contributes to emotional stability and a positive mental attitude."

Wouldn't it be amazing if a new generation of broth converts improved not only their own health but that of their children? Imagine how good everyone would feel, with brains and bodies working in optimal harmony. Imagine how much better students would concentrate and learn if they weren't being given processed, GMO-ridden food for school breakfasts and lunches. Think how much more effective our soldiers would be if their rations were wholesome. Envision how much better the rehabilitation of our inmates in the prison system would be if their meals were healthy.

Broth isn't just the fountain of youth. Making broth for yourself and your loved ones is an investment in your future. With only a few minutes of effort, you will reap enormous rewards.

NOTE: It is extremely important that these broths are made with the right kind of bones, or they will be lacking in many of the essential micronutrients your body craves. This means that the healthiest broth comes from organically raised, grass-fed animals, without any use of hormones, antibiotics, pesticides, or herbicides. Not even "grain-finished"—this is a sneaky way of cutting costs where the label says "grass-fed," but in fact the animals were fed grass for only a certain period of time, then switched to hormone-ridden feed at the end. Be an informed consumer; it's really okay to become that inquisitive person at the counter asking if the bones are only grain-finished or fully grass-fed. Always seek to buy bones from a reputable organic source, either in person or online.

THE IMPORTANCE OF
Collagen

COLLAGEN IS THE MOST ABUNDANT PROTEIN in the human body. (Approximately 25 to 35 percent of protein is collagen.) Regarded as the substance that holds the whole body together, collagen can be found in the bones, muscles, skin, and tendons. It allows for movement, agility, flexibility, and expansion in all these parts of your body. Collagen helps your fascia (remember that word from Chapter 1—it's the connective tissue under our skin) to be long, lean, and flexible, to make your body strong and supple.

Collagen plays many roles in the body, in three different categories:

AESTHETIC COLLAGEN

We all want to be as attractive and sexy as possible. Aesthetic collagen is the collagen responsible for the healthy skin, hair, and nails that make us look foxy. The more collagen you have, the slower the aging process, internally and externally (no wonder collagen is such a buzzword in the beauty industry!).

FITNESS COLLAGEN

Athletes all over the world know that the more flexible their joints and bones are, the less likely they are to get injured. Collagen is the secret to well-lubricated, well-cushioned joints and spinal cord.

Remember the plastic model of a spinal cord hanging in the corner of your high school biology classroom? It was usually made with pieces of rubber sandwiched between the vertebrae, representing the real disks of the spine that cushion the vertebrae. These disks are primarily composed of collagen, so a diet lacking in it due to GMOs and processed food is directly correlated to herniated (or slipped) disks and other back issues, all of which are extremely painful and limit your range of motion.

You need broth to lubricate your joints. When weekend warriors exercise full-bore after working long hours at their mostly sedentary jobs during the week, they are susceptible to injuries of the rotator cuff and shoulders, knees, elbows, and lower back. These types of injuries are far less prevalent in cultures where broth is a regular part of the diet. Older people remain active and healthy, and they are revered for their sage advice. In our American culture now, unfortunately, our older generations are being hit with early onset degenerative diseases, and information that molds the next generation is not being passed down.

There's no reason to hear yourself saying, "Oh, it's just the way it is," or "My bones are creaking because I'm getting older," when broth can provide the rejuvenation you've been seeking. Elizabeth has seen this with her clients who are athletes; their tennis elbow, sore knees and shoulders, and aches and pains go away.

INTERNAL HEALTH COLLAGEN

Broth expert Sally Fallon explained that our intestines are made of a sort of skin, which as you previously learned contains a thick layer of collagen. "GMOs cause holes to form in the skin of our guts," she explained, which allows waste to escape through them and into your system. "The collagen in broth helps to repair these holes." This prevents the evil invaders from leaching out into our blood, leading to an array of issues, such as toxicity, autoimmune disorders, and inflammation.

It's Elizabeth's theory that the lack of collagen in our blood is leading to the autoimmune diseases that afflict so many people now, much as Laura suffered from Hashimoto's thyroiditis, which affected her thyroid function. My goal is to help reverse this trend. After all, autoimmune issues arise from the outside in, so try healing from the inside out with bone broth—allowing you to do your utmost to reverse by replenishing.

LAURA

I've never had any work done to my face, so imagine my surprise when I opened up one of those tabloid magazines recently to find some doctor (who has never treated me, of course) claiming that I'd had a brow lift, a nose job, and fillers in my face because of how much the "tone" of my face has improved. My face looks so much more luminous and smooth now than it did several years ago, yet the only difference in that time? I've been working with Elizabeth and following the Stash Plan. In particular, I've been drinking my daily bone broth, full of that beautiful collagen. It really is the fountain of youth!

ELIZABETH

After my daughter was born, I breast-fed her for two years. Women in my studio couldn't believe that I didn't have stretch marks. The collagen in my body was different from theirs because of the food I was eating. If your body is being fed good broth and other foods, allowing it to heal while you're losing weight, you shouldn't have a major problem with stretch marks.

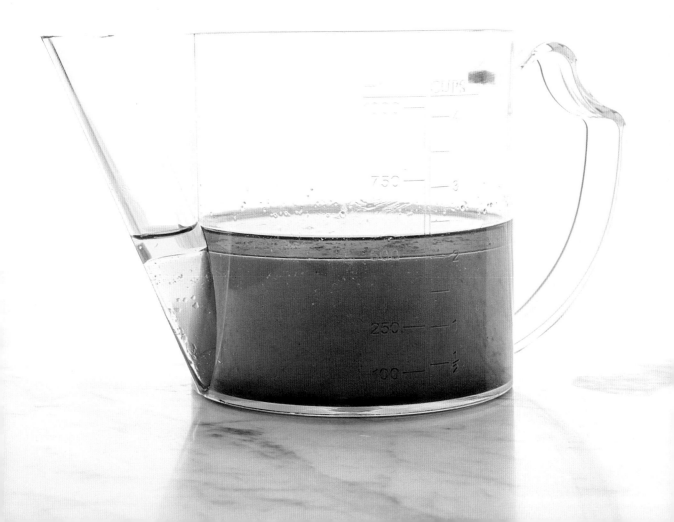

BONES

People take for granted that you can get out of bed and walk, but without bones, you wouldn't be any more stable than a jellyfish. Bones in broth are not there just for flavor—they're the literal essence of the broth. That's because bone tissue is primarily made from connective tissue (your collagen) and calcium!

If, however, you don't have the mineral content your body needs, your body will pull it from somewhere. It looks to the bones and starts to leach the minerals out of them, causing them to become more fragile and brittle. Over time, this leads to what is called osteoporosis.

Keep your bones strong by drinking broth. Ronaldo Ferraris, a researcher at the New Jersey Medical School of Rutgers, has concluded that fructose (derived from corn and sugar cane) inhibits the intestine's absorption of calcium, which results in fragile bones. Athletes should shun

• • • • • • • • • • • **LAURA** • • • • • • • • • • •

Sometimes I'll be talking to one of my best friends and ask what she did the previous night, and she'll say, "I ate a pint of Ben and Jerry's, felt so gross about myself, then passed out. Why did I do this to myself when I know better?" We've all asked ourselves this question and can relate in some way. Why are we compelled to do something we know we shouldn't? Like eating an entire bag of chips or three doughnuts or going for another heaping serving when you know you're full. It's not just a lack of willpower.

Another aspect is emotional eating. It tends to come on suddenly and usually is attached to specific cravings for comfort food—and it can become addictive. We also tend to overindulge in the foods that may lead to us feeling powerless, guilty, or shameful. Interestingly, in Chinese Meridian Theory, "addiction" and "the deepest emotion" are housed in the liver, as well as "appetite" and "overeating." Naturally, as you follow the Stash Plan and get your liver working at a higher capacity, bad habits will be replaced with good habits. Your sudden urges, cravings, and addictions will even out and diminish.

sports drinks loaded with fructose and drink bone broth and water instead. This would naturally lead to fewer injuries.

In fact, in a January 22, 2015, *Washington Post* article basketball star Kobe Bryant admitted that bone broths not only helped him recover from injuries but improved his overall health and playing ability.

CARTILAGE

Cartilage is flexible connective tissue—it's what ears and noses are made of. (Li'l fun fact: Ears and noses are the only two body parts that never stop growing, due to cartilage cells continuing to divide as we get older. So yes, your grandparents really do have bigger noses and ears!) When you cook bones in water to make broth, the cartilage disintegrates. This is exactly what you want, and you'll know you've cooked your broth properly when it solidifies into gelatin when it becomes cold. This melted-down cartilage is part of what makes broth so healthy, as it strengthens your own cartilage, joints, and bones.

BONE MARROW

Marrow is the soft tissue found inside bones that creates our blood cells, as well as the lymphocytes so necessary for a strong immune system to protect against foreign invaders. It comes in red and yellow. Red marrow is responsible for the creation of red and white blood cells; the average adult's marrow produces over 500 *billion* new red blood cells every day. Yellow marrow is your body's storehouse for fats and aids the immune system in killing off pathogens.

Healthy bone marrow makes for healthy bodies. If you eat foods you now know you shouldn't, eventually, as with Laura, toxins can overwhelm your lymphatic system. Once there, they can compromise your immune system in many ways, leading to autoimmune disorders and increased susceptibility to colds and flus.

Fortunately, adding broth to your daily diet will build your defenses and help your body's constitution change into a strong fighting machine!

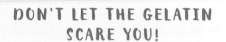

DON'T LET THE GELATIN SCARE YOU!

Meat gelatin, which is mostly made of collagen, might look a bit strange when you take your Stash container out of the fridge, but it melts into an amazing tonic when it's heated.

Gelatin is not a complete protein, but it acts as a protein "sparer," allowing the broth protein to be saved and dispersed to keep you on an even keel throughout the day—as opposed to spiking, then crashing, as is true of those who eat a lot of foods containing refined sugars and complex white carbohydrates. If, for instance, you tend to get very hungry and craving sugary carbs at three or four p.m.—the time that many people do, after their lunch has digested and not provided enough nutrition for their starving cells—try drinking broth instead. It's soothing and filling even though it's very low in calories.

In fact, broths are actually the original fast food. A pot would be left simmering on the stove or fire all day, and whatever other ingredients were available would be added to it to make a complete meal. You can do this with your Stashes. Veggies that are starting to wilt, for example, can get tossed into the soup pot with the bones, and this will make an ever more nutritious tonic.

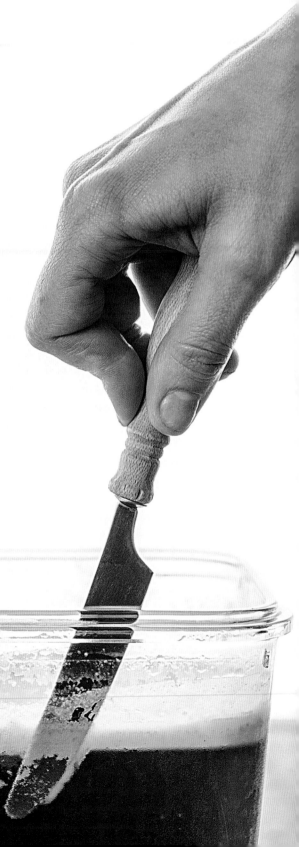

ALL ABOUT
Glutamine

COLLAGEN IS A LARGE PROTEIN MOLECULE made up of over a thousand amino acids. Among them are arginine (improving blood flow to enhance circulation) and glycine (for internal growth and strong bones). Most important of all is glutamine.

Think of glutamine as the foundation for all the other amino acids; they need glutamine to ignite them, like having a great coach rallying the team to the state championship. Glutamine strengthens your immune system. It helps the small intestine villi to heal and grow, allowing for optimal absorption of nutrients; this will ultimately lead to less hunger as your body will be properly nourished. It promotes production of new skin cells, so it can slow down the aging process, helping your skin stay firm and strong; this is why it's often referred to as the "internal fountain of youth." Glutamine is also intrinsic to muscle growth, and many body builders take supplements regularly. They know that long cardio or weight-training sessions—as well as daily stressors—drain your body of glutamine faster than you can replenish it. When that happens, glutamine is pulled out of the muscles for energy. Bone broth replenishes it.

Glutamine and Your Brain

Glutamine is also a brain food, meaning that it can cross the blood-brain barrier (BBB) into your actual brain tissue. The BBB is like a force field protecting the brain from foreign substances that may injure it; it protects the brain from hormones and neurotransmitters in the rest of the body; and it maintains the necessary environment so these functions can thrive. The BBB is semipermeable; it allows only some materials to cross. Getting the micronutrients you need to cross the BBB is not easy!

Chemicals from food and/or the environment break down the BBB. "Junk food" is a term used for foods containing high levels of calories from sugar, simple carbohydrates, and/or fat, with little or no protein, fiber, vitamins, and/or minerals. Wonder Bread, the top seller in America, is junk food, as it's made from highly processed GMO wheat flour, soybean oil, high-fructose corn syrup, and sodium stearoyl lactylate—an ingredient similar to what's found in Styrofoam.

For example, many Americans start their day with a bowl of processed and fortified sweetened cereal. Honey Nut Cheerios is number one, and number two is Frosted Flakes, which contains a whopping thirty grams of sugar in each cup—and most people eat much more than that. This type of food breaks down the BBB, leading to attention span and mood disorders in many children, and brain fog, irritability, and memory retention problems in adults. Broth, however, has a positive effect on *all* this potential BBB breakdown. Although most Americans don't consider broth a breakfast food, many cultures do, particularly in Asia. Try swapping your sweet cereal for nourishing bone broth for a few days while on the Stash Plan, and you'll be amazed by the results.

Often consumers think some food items are healthy due to marketing and packaging. (A perfect example of this is a protein bar, usually chockfull of GMO soy and sugars.) The more junk food a person eats, the more a person tends to crave it—but you're not completely to blame for this. Countless millions of dollars are spent by food manufacturers on understanding the physical and psychological cravings for junk food so that consumers readily succumb to that perfect crunch of a chip, the quintessential fizz of a soda after you pop open a can, or the classic golden-yellow color of a Twinkie.

"Big Food" scientists are paid to learn what makes people want more; food manufacturers are calculatedly banking, literally, on our being addicted to these foods. Experiments show that the same reward and pleasure centers of the brain that are triggered by drugs such as cocaine and heroin are also activated by food—particularly food high in sugar, fat, and salt. The feel-good brain chemicals such as dopamine override other signals telling your brain that you're full or satisfied, so you keep eating even when you're not truly hungry anymore.

The Collagen Connection and Your Fascia

As you know, the primary component of bone broth is collagen. The same goes for fascia. Not only that, but the composition of beef, chicken, and fish broth is an almost identical mimic of the 3-D web of gluey wet proteins of your fascia. When fascia is not gnarled up, it resembles a cheesecloth-like grid and is smooth. Ideally, it's a thin layer surrounding the muscles.

When you consistently replenish your body's fascia with the good kind of fascia found in bone broth, this allows your energy to flow through it effortlessly. This is what makes muscles longer and leaner.

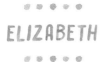

ELIZABETH

When a person's fascia is a maze of gnarled and stuck knots, it makes them either totally numb or totally in pain. Either you feel nothing, as Laura did, or you're so sensitive to the touch that it's unbearable. Even though Laura and I did aggressive stretching, she had no recovery pain. Through ongoing sessions of Thai massage, I started to release deeper fascia in her quadriceps. Once her fascia started to smooth out and pull away from dense muscle tissue, she regained her strength and power—and she also lost weight and became much leaner.

Four Different Broths

1. BEEF BROTH

After so many years of making broth, we believe that beef broth is the "backbone" of all broths. It is what you sip when you need to feel grounded and stable, as it gives you strength and stamina. Of all the broths, it contains the most marrow and collagen. Cancel the Botox party, and make it a bone broth party instead!

2. CHICKEN BROTH

Chicken broth is an immune booster and a healing modality in many cultures.

Everybody loves it, from young children to the elderly. Its mild flavor makes it easy to incorporate into many recipes, making it not only delicious but practical.

3. FISH BROTH

An extremely common deficiency in the American diet is of omega 3 and 6 essential fatty acids, or EFAs, needed for the essential functioning of all your body's tissues. Your body can't make them, so you need to get them either through a good diet or via supplements (usually fish oil). In addition, EFAs need to be taken in the proper ratio. When you make fish broth, the fish already has the perfect balance. Fish broth is also ideal for brainpower and focus.

An excellent add-on option for fish broth is seaweed. Seaweeds are rich in antioxidants, calcium, and iodine (which supports the thyroid in regulating hormones). As you've read already, the liver is one of the body's organs that manufactures hormones, so a seaweed-enriched broth enables the liver and thyroid to work as a team.

If you're a bit leery of the smell, it does help to make this broth in a slow cooker, but the aroma really isn't overwhelming. Fish broth is delicate and delicious.

4. VEGETABLE BROTH

Although the nutrients extracted from meat or fish bones aren't a component of vegetable broths, our recipes are still highly nutritious and suitable for vegetarians and vegans. Adding a bit of seaweed is also a good option.

We'll give you detailed recipes for each of these four essential broths in Chapter 10. But man (or woman) cannot live on broth alone! (That sounds dangerously close to one of those crash diets that the Stash Plan is the exact opposite of!) You'll be eating plenty of real, delicious food, so read on to Chapter 6 to learn the basic components of food on the Stash Plan.

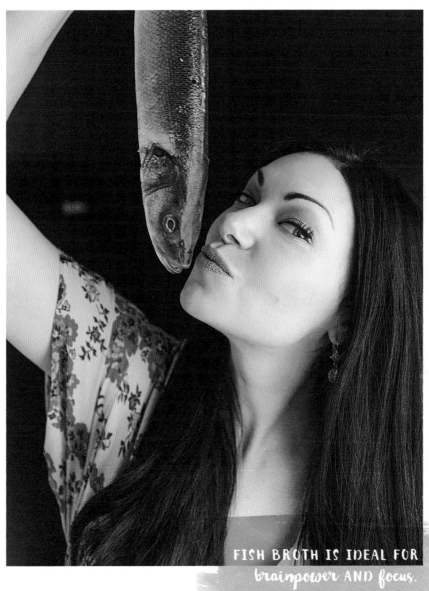

FISH BROTH IS IDEAL FOR *brainpower* AND *focus.*

REAL

Food YOU CAN Take

ANYWHERE

chapter 6

The Digestive Duo of your gallbladder and liver have been relentless in their battles, constantly working to keep you healthy, so now it's time to take care of them. They come home from a long day of crime-fighting and digesting, and they need dinner on the table and their feet rubbed as well. Foods with high amounts of antioxidants, good fats, and fiber help our duo replenish what they've expended through their trials and tribulations of dealing with what we've eaten.

LET'S START WITH ANTIOXIDANTS.

The Importance of
ANTIOXIDANTS

"OXIDATION IS A VERY NATURAL PROCESS that happens during normal cellular function," says Jeffrey Blumberg, a professor of nutrition at Tufts University in Boston. You've seen oxidation in action when an apple slice turns brown, a bike left out in the rain get rusty, or a cut on your skin develops a scab. Antioxidant literally means no oxygen, so it makes sense that antioxidants are compounds that counteract the effects of oxidation, which takes place when a cell or a substance loses electrons and undergoes changes as a result. The cells either die (the apple shrivels) or are replaced with new cells (the scab). When your body is not functioning normally—especially when it's being fed GMO-tainted food or other unhealthy things—the rate of cellular damage can increase.

Antioxidants equal antiaging. When a cell is damaged, it releases free radicals, unstable molecules that have lost an electron and will do anything to replace it—mainly by poaching electrons from other cells, damaging the new cells, and allowing the cycle to continue. This is called oxidative stress. Some diseases associated with oxidative stress are all cancers, diabetes, cardiovascular disease, Alzheimer's, and Parkinson's.

Fortunately, antioxidants fight and neutralize free radicals, then heal the damaged area of the cell. You want as many of them patrolling your body as possible, ferreting out the free radicals and destroying them. One of the most kick-ass antioxidants is glutathione.

Made in the liver, glutathione is a master detoxifier. Let's think of it as one of the stars of *Law & Order*, racing to the scene to catch the bad guys in the middle of a crime spree. In *our* show, antioxidants like glutathione use sulfur as their weapon of choice to pull in free radicals, heavy metals, viruses, and bacteria, and destroy them so your lymphatic system can ship them out. Sulfur should be the third most abundant mineral in the body, after calcium and phosphorus (the minerals that keep our bones and teeth strong), and we get it almost entirely through what we eat. But many of us

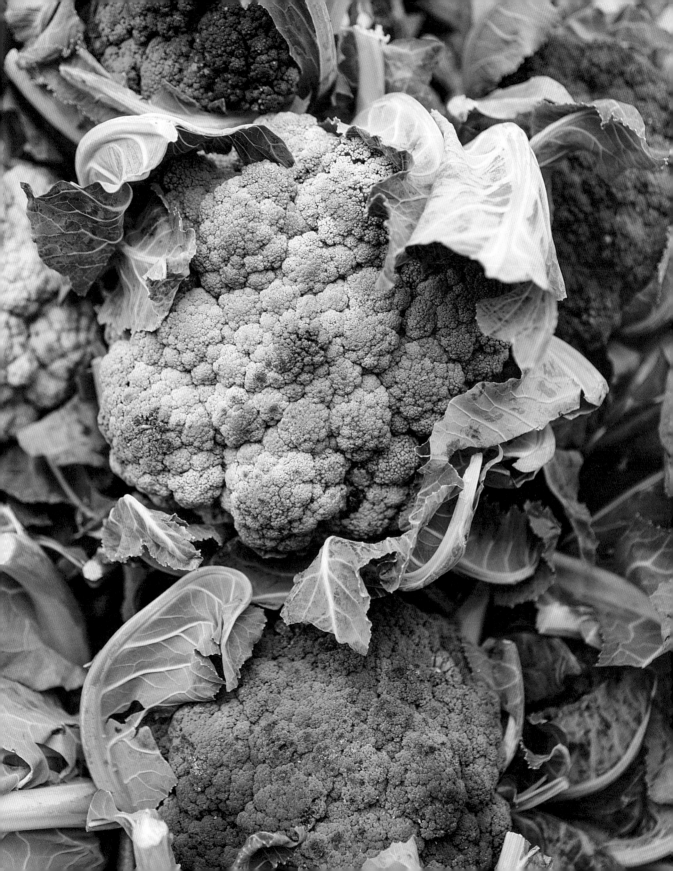

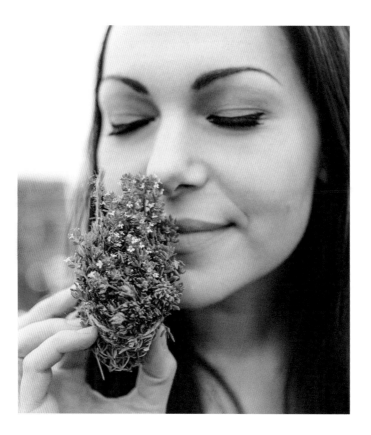

are sulfur-depleted thanks to the damage done to the soil our food grows in. Pesticides, herbicides, and overfarming deplete our soil of nutrients, making the crops sulfur-deficient. A lot of vegetables with a strong, pungent smell are loaded with sulfur: brussels sprouts, cabbage, garlic, onions (sulfur is what brings tears to your eyes when you cut it), and parsnips. A sulfur deficiency is one of the culprits for many age-related problems—that's why it's considered the "beauty mineral."

Eating foods with high levels of glutathione and other antioxidants will make you stronger and more resilient in response to the environmental stressors in the world around you and inside of you. (It's always better to eat your nutrients than to take them as supplements, which might not be processed properly by your body. Especially if your liver and gallbladder are already overtaxed, as most of ours are.) As we know, in our modern world, it is almost impossible to avoid environmental toxins. We drive cars, we live in cities stifled with smog, we spray our crops with pesticides and herbicides, and we live near power plants. What is done in one country affects those in neighboring countries, as pollutants get into the water and the air. There is a constant ripple effect. On an enormous level, if a large factory is spewing toxic waste, that affects all nearby cities or towns. On a smaller level, if you're spraying your lawn with what you think is a harmless weed killer but is actually glyphosate, you could be putting your neighbors at risk.

THE BEST WAYS TO KEEP YOUR LIVER PRODUCING OPTIMUM AMOUNTS OF GLUTATHIONE

- Eat organic produce. It's pricier, yes. But it really does make a difference, for all the reasons we've discussed in this book. We have all seen the difference in price between organic and nonorganic foods. The reasons to invest in organic foods are the same reason to put the highest level of gasoline in your car; it runs better and lasts longer and performs better! Organic foods are filled with micronutrients and are vibrantly alive. They feed your body in a way that make you feel energized and satisfied. Nonorganic foods fill you up, but then an hour later you are wanting more food. This is because your body craves the nutrition, not the bulk! Some of the more affordable options for organic foods are farmers' markets, food co-ops, or a backyard garden (if you're lucky enough to have the space for such a thing). And be sure to pay special attention to the annual "Organic Dirty Dozen"—a list put out each year by the Environmental Working Group

ELIZABETH

I was living in upstate New York at the time and got a gorgeous eight-week-old puppy named Cooper for my daughter on her tenth birthday. He loved to play on my neighbor's lawn, but started having seizures after a few weeks. I realized it was because my neighbors were having their lawn sprayed with weed killers every Monday morning. I believe the chemicals in the sprays got into Cooper's central nervous system, affecting his brain activity, as he sniffed around with his nose, ate the grass, and rolled around on it. Now imagine babies and kids playing on lawns sprayed with these same chemicals and how this could dangerously affect their delicate, growing bodies. We want the Stash Plan to help you fend off anything that can damage your body, so you can live a happy and healthy life.

of the fruits and vegetables that are typically the most contaminated and that you should try to prioritize eating organic.

- Eat antioxidant-rich vegetables such as avocados, cruciferous vegetables (broccoli, cabbage, cauliflower), garlic, kale, onions, parsley, parsnips, radish, squashes, tomatoes, turnips, and watercress.

- Avoid processed foods. Basically, anything man has altered.

- Maintain healthy exercise—and allow plenty of time for recovery. Glutathione production is dependent on ATP (adenosine triphosphate, the energy currency of your cells). Exercise such as rebounding, swimming, power walking, and stretching all produce the most ATP in the body. Ironically, exceedingly strenuous exercise causes the opposite—an extreme drop in ATP that leads to free radical production and cellular damage.

- Enjoy raw milk, raw eggs, and raw cheese. All three increase glutathione production as long as they are raw; pasteurization destroys it. Find a trustworthy local farm through the Weston A. Price Foundation or www.realmilk.com.

- Eat organic grass-fed meats and organ meats. For the same reasons it's vital to use organic, grass-fed bones for your bone broth—these foods regenerate glutathione in your body.

- Cook with organic turmeric. This bright orange spice supports the liver in filtering blood and detoxification, which helps raise glutathione levels.

- Incorporate lots of garlic and onions into your diet. Garlic is the *best* food for your gallbladder and liver. It detoxes these organs as well as your blood, and contains high levels of sulfur. And all varieties of onions are high in glutathione. Onions also lower blood pressure and cholesterol, and they are antiviral, helping to reduce symptoms of the common cold.

- Explore ume plum vinegar. Ume plum vinegar is high in antioxidants and it aids in digestion, helping the body assimilate nutrients.

Additional Potent Antioxidants

Consider these antioxidants the supporting roles to our leading man, glutathione:

ALPHA-LIPOIC ACID (ALA): THE BRAIN ANTIOXIDANT

This is the Watson to Sherlock Holmes.

ALA is the only antioxidant that can easily be transported through the BBB to the brain, where it helps with memory and mental focus. It is an excellent anti-inflammatory, a great free radical scavenger, and a potent heavy metal chelator (pulls heavy metals from the blood). ALA has the ability to regenerate/recycle other antioxidants like vitamins C and E as well as glutathione. Another important function of ALA is that it converts food to energy.

Foods that contain ALA: beets, brewer's yeast, brussels sprouts, carrots, fennel, dried red beans, organ meats (heart, liver, kidneys), peas, potatoes, rice bran, spinach.

COENZYME Q10 (COQ10): THE HEART ANTIOXIDANT

This is the Lois to Clark Kent.

CoQ10 has many functions. It protects the heart from free radicals, helps maintain normal blood pressure, reduces signs of aging, helps your cells produce more energy, and helps keep your nervous system running smoothly.

Foods that contain CoQ10: berries, such as blackberries and wild blueberries—the darker the fruit, the more antioxidants it contains; cold-pressed organic oils; fatty fish, such as wild-caught organic salmon, tuna, and herring; organic beef and chicken; peanuts; pistachios, sesame seeds.

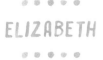

ELIZABETH The demand for organic is high, and just like anything it will get to a tipping point and then changes will happen. They are already starting to happen! I was in a natural food store the other day and I saw organic grass-fed bones for $5.99. Which is a huge difference from what it was when I started making broths.

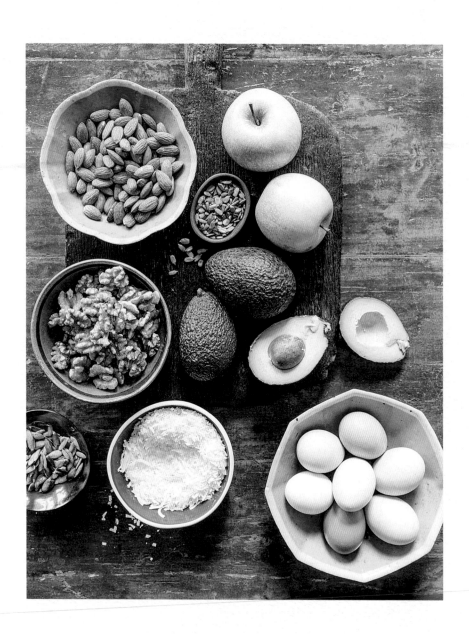

ASTAXANTHIN, CAROTENOIDS, AND RESVERATROL: THE FEEL-GOOD ANTIOXIDANTS

These are the fairy godmothers to Cinderella.

This trio of antioxidants can all lower blood pressure, inhibit the spread of cancers, and help prevent Alzheimer's disease. Astaxanthin is extremely beneficial as it contains twenty times more antioxidants than carotenoids, which are found in the foods that put color on your plate. Resveratrol is found in foods with jewel tones, like purple and deep red.

Foods that contain astaxanthin: algae, crab, krill, lobster, rainbow trout, shrimp, sockeye salmon; it's found in the flesh and bones. These fish should always be wild-caught because they contain 400 percent more astaxanthin than farm-raised fish and seafood.

Foods that contain carotenoids: beet greens, cabbage, carrots, collard greens, kale, pumpkin, spinach, turnip greens, sweet potatoes, winter squash.

Foods that contain resveratrol: blueberries, bilberries, cranberries, grapes, lingonberries, mulberries.

A Few Words about Fats

NOT ALL FATS are created equal. Fats to be aware of:

- Saturated fats create energy and fuel for your body, and they are primarily found in animal sources such as dairy, eggs, meat, and poultry. Saturated fats have been seen as unhealthy for decades, starting in the 1950s, when they were blamed for clogged arteries, high blood pressure and weight gain. In truth, what's most dangerous about these fats is how they are processed and used in cooking, and if the body is capable of breaking them correctly. It's best to use coconut oil, which is a saturated fat laden with health benefits.

- Trans fats are bad fats. *Trans* is a Latin prefix meaning across or beyond, and trans fats do just that—taking food beyond what it should naturally be by extending its shelf life and keeping it "fresh" for extended periods of time.

BUTTER IS BETTER THAN MARGARINE!

Butter is made from cream and is a *real* food recognized by your body. Margarine, on the other hand, is made from hydrogenated and refined vegetable, soy, corn, and/or cottonseed oil, which as you know are at the top of the GMO list in Chapter 4. Many consumers erroneously think that margarine is more heart healthy than butter, but they're wrong. Margarine actually causes weight gain and cholesterol because it's so highly processed that the liver can't recognize it, so it's stored as fat instead.

Trans fats raise bad cholesterol levels and lower good cholesterol levels, and they also cause circulatory issues and create aging in the body. They're found in packaged baked goods such as cakes, cookies, and pies; in snacks like corn chips and potato chips; in foods that require deep frying (French fries, doughnuts, fried chicken); in margarine; and in nondairy creamers.

Monounsaturated fats cleanse the body of acids while fueling metabolism. Avocados, olive oil, and nuts such as almonds, macadamias, cashews, and pecans have the highest levels. Olive and avocado oils are ideal for cooking because they can withstand heat above 118 degrees; high heat can chemically transform other good oils into trans fats.

- Polyunsaturated fats (omega 3 and 6) neutralize acids that can cause damage to your heart and brain; the more acid, the more free radicals. They also help your arteries stay clear of bad cholesterol. Salmon, sunflower seeds, and walnuts are the foods most rich in polyunsaturated fats.

LAURA

As you read earlier in the book, I tried one low-fat diet after another when I was struggling with my weight, each one contradicting the other and leading to more and more problems. When I finally realized that low-fat diets don't work and instead started eating to fuel and nourish my body with real fats, my body was finally able to start letting go of unwanted pounds. I wasn't tricking it into thinking it was starving anymore.

A Few Words about Fiber

FIBER INTAKE affects all aspects of the digestive process, especially as it pulls waste products out of the large intestine so it can be eliminated. It also absorbs excess bile, sponges up the pathogens the blood is trying to get rid of, and helps prevent heart attacks because it soaks up toxins so they're not recycled back to your heart.

Fiber is either soluble (can be dissolved in water) or insoluble (doesn't break down in water). There is a reason for both. Soluble fiber gets absorbed into the blood, which keeps blood sugar stable so your energy levels don't spike up and down. Insoluble fiber works as a sponge, pulling bad toxins from the blood and unwanted solid waste from the intestines. This helps to speed up the elimination of waste from your body as it keeps you regular.

Foods that contain high levels of fiber: apples (especially the peel), artichokes, beets, berries, broccoli, cabbage, carrots, cauliflower, celery, dark leafy greens, dried beans, grapefruit, lentils, mushrooms, oranges, seeds, squashes, and tropical fruits.

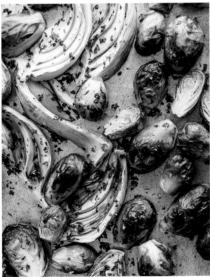 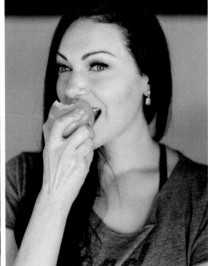

Beneficial Drinks

IN GENERAL, water is the best choice for everybody. But you can't always just drink water, as there are so many other beverages that can quench your thirst and tickle your taste buds. It's very helpful to know that there are liquids as beneficial for your gallbladder and liver as the foods you'll eat.

- Almond milk. It's incredibly easy to make your own nut milk—you just have to remember to soak the nuts overnight. Look for the recipe on page 230. We love lattes made with homemade almond milk, which helps break down saturated fats.

- Apple cider. A satisfying drink is one with ¼ cup cider to ½ cup seltzer.

- Apple cider vinegar. A terrific tonic is to drink one tablespoon of raw organic apple cider vinegar in eight ounces of water every day. Apple cider vinegar works as a natural antifungal (great for the gallbladder), as a natural antibiotic, and as an antiseptic to fight germs and bacteria before they get to your liver.

- Beet juice. It creates new blood in the liver and keeps your gallbladder dumping its bile properly. Try mixing it with ice water or seltzer with a bit of lime and/or orange squeezed in.

- Coffee, always organic. The caffeine and other compounds in coffee are stimulating while breaking down fat and curbing your appetite. Just not too much, and not all day long, like Laura used to do.

- Ginger tea. Hot or cold ginger tea helps break down high-protein foods; it neutralizes uric acid from eating a high-protein animal diet.

LAURA

I absolutely love nuts! My friends nicknamed me Squirrel and even bought me a little squirrel statue I keep next to my stove. One thing I love to do is to soak raw nuts, especially almonds, in water or pineapple juice until they're soft—they soak up the enzymes from the juice and become even more nutritious—and then I put these on salads and make trail mixes. This is a great substitute for roasted nuts if you are sensitive to them like I tend to be.

- Green tea, either iced or hot, with lots of lemon. LAURA: I like to add some powdered matcha green tea to my regular green tea. It gives it that vibrant green color and boosts up the flavor and antioxidants.

- Kombucha. This drink is an anticoagulant for blood as well as a natural fungicide.

- Lemon juice, fresh squeezed. It's especially great first thing in the morning. Your liver does all its heavy-duty detox in the middle of the night, which makes your stomach acidic—so the cooling nature of lemon juice helps neutralize stomach acid. It's the most valuable fruit for anyone who's eaten a high-fat meal the night before.

  In addition, when your gallbladder and liver aren't functioning well, your saliva changes and speeds along the deterioration of your gums and teeth. Lemons neutralize saliva, cleanse the gums, and purify bacteria lurking in your mouth with their astringent properties. They also flush out inflammation from lymph nodes, lessen the production of mucus, encourage the formation of bile, improve mineral absorption, lower blood pressure, and promote healthy blood circulation.

  So drink up the lemon water! We like to use one whole lemon per eight-ounce glass of water. The more you drink it, the more you'll crave it. Just try to use a straw to drink the pure lemon water, because the only downside to it is that it can break down the enamel on your teeth.

Beneficial Herbs and Vitamins

YOU CAN ALSO USE different herbs and vitamins to keep your gallbladder and liver in great shape. Look for these:

- B complex. It helps with the formation of red blood cells.

- B6. It stimulates the gallbladder and helps break down gallstones.

- Basil. This vibrant herb detoxes the blood.

- Black pepper. It stimulates digestion and opens up your pores for more efficient sweating and detoxing.

- Cilantro. This aromatic herb is a powerful in chelating blood (pulling toxins and heavy metals from the bloodstream). Cilantro opens energy to the brain stem, which allows you to think clearly; this makes it particularly beneficial for children living with autism spectrum issues or for the elderly with forms of dementia. Use cilantro in drinks and as a pesto sauce so you can eat as much of it as possible at one meal. Adding fresh chopped cilantro to your dishes will also make you look and feel like a gourmet chef!

- Dill. It's calming for digestion and is great at dissolving mucus.

- Garlic. This is the best thing for your liver—it detoxes not just this organ but your blood, too.

- Horseradish. If you've ever tried it, you know it clears your sinuses right up, and is also an antiparasitic.

- Lecithin granules. They provide mono-unsaturated fat, are easily digested, cleanse the body of acids, and aid in metabolism. It doesn't hurt that they're also a great brain food. They can be found in most natural food stores.

YOU CAN USE A VARIETY OF *herbs and vitamins* TO KEEP YOUR GALLBLADDER AND LIVER IN *great shape.*

- Milk thistle. It repairs and rejuvenates the liver, and actually helps it grow more new cells. Li'l fun fact: Milk thistle after a night of partying helps with hangovers the next day.

- Turmeric. This bright yellow herb is one of the most potent anti-inflammatories you can take.

- Vitamins A, C, E, and D. These vitamins are antioxidants and help neutralize free radicals.

Support Your Inner Cravings

EVERYBODY KNOWS what it's like to have cravings! These alternatives are an excellent way to manage those impulsive cravings that can jam up your gallbladder and liver. As always, make sure your new choices are organic.

	PUSH IT AWAY	STASHIFY
Main Dishes	Fast-food burger	Grass-fed Sliders
	Fried chicken	Coconut Almond Chicken
	Pasta, white flour	Cilantro Pesto Brown Rice Noodles
	French fries	Herb-Roasted Sweet Potato Home Fries
	Taco Bell	Turmeric Turkey
	Hamburger Helper Three Cheese	Pot Roast and Yucca Pucks
	Canned soup	Nutrient-packed life force bone broth
Side Dishes	Cup noodles	Quinoa Tabbouleh
	Rice-A-Roni	Purple Rice Stir-fry
	Instant/powdered mashed potatoes	Mashed Cauliflower
	Bagged Dole insta-salad	Salad Shakers
	Wonder Bread grilled cheese	Avocado, butter-toasted Gluten-Free Almond Bread

You should never go hungry on the Stash Plan. There is so much to keep you satiated and help your liver and gallbladder to flourish and burn fat to their highest potential!

In Chapter 9, we'll take you through the preparation, cooking, and storage of one complete Stash—in other words, three days of delicious meals. And you'll also learn how to pack up your meals and take them with you, wherever you need to go. Then in Chapter 11 we'll give you the recipes for five more Stashes, so you'll have plenty of variety in your menus. But first let's look at the third pillar of the Stash Plan—muscle meridian stretching.

Energize THROUGH STRETCHING

chapter 7

Most people think of stretching as something to do before or after a workout to warm up or cool down their muscles and joints—grabbing your ankle and pulling it up to your glutes to stretch your quadriceps muscle, for example; or kicking your foot up onto something and leaning forward to stretch your hamstrings. The Stash Plan stretches are very different.

The Muscle Meridian Method (M3) developed by Elizabeth is a stretching and strengthening technique that fires an energy pathway to a specific organ, and when this happens, it helps a person physically as well as psychologically. Basically, with M3, when you resist in the stretch, the meridian fires through the muscle, which then affects the function of the correlated organ. This is the same concept as acupuncture, where a very fine needle is inserted at various points of the body, which in turn fires the related meridian.

Kenny Florian, former elite Ultimate Fighting Championship fighter and current host of *UFC Tonight*, had this to say about M3: "Because I trust Laura's knowledge when it comes to health and nutrition I agreed to work with Elizabeth Troy and see how she could help me optimize my body to perform at its peak state. Elizabeth showed me some amazing stretching positions and techniques that immediately made me feel better, and gave me a plan to turn my weaknesses and imbalances into strengths. Elizabeth's knowledge about the human body was so impressive, and the results I got from her made me a true believer in her methods. I wish I had known these things when I was competing."

Another remarkable aspect of Chinese Meridian Theory and M3 is that the gallbladder and liver are always the *start* of the energy cycle. When you get these meridians opened, the other organ functions will improve as well.

Why M3 Stretching
IS SO EFFECTIVE

Firing the Gallbladder Meridian

According to Chinese Meridian Theory, the main gallbladder meridian runs up the outside of the leg into the side of your booty, where the main trigger point called Gallbladder 30 is located, then continues up to the side of the forehead. Breaking up the fascia around the Gallbladder 30 trigger point to open up meridian flow will cause fat-burning to become more efficient. This is the smallest organ and the largest meridian.

Firing the Liver Meridian

The main meridian for the liver runs up the inside of the leg and the lateral muscles on the sides of your back. When you fire these meridians, your legs get longer and leaner, and your lateral muscles shift shape, giving you a much more defined V-shape in your rib cage and a smaller waist.

In some extreme cases, these blocked meridians and constricted muscle groups are so over-tightened as to cause people to walk with their feet turned out. Conversely, you've probably seen people walk pigeon-toed, with their toes turned in; this too is often due to muscles being so tightly constricted that the legs are pulled in toward each other.

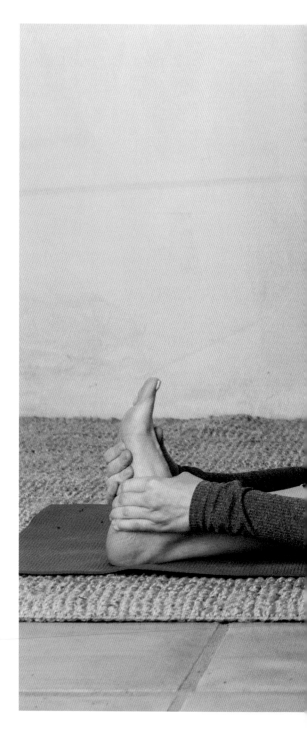

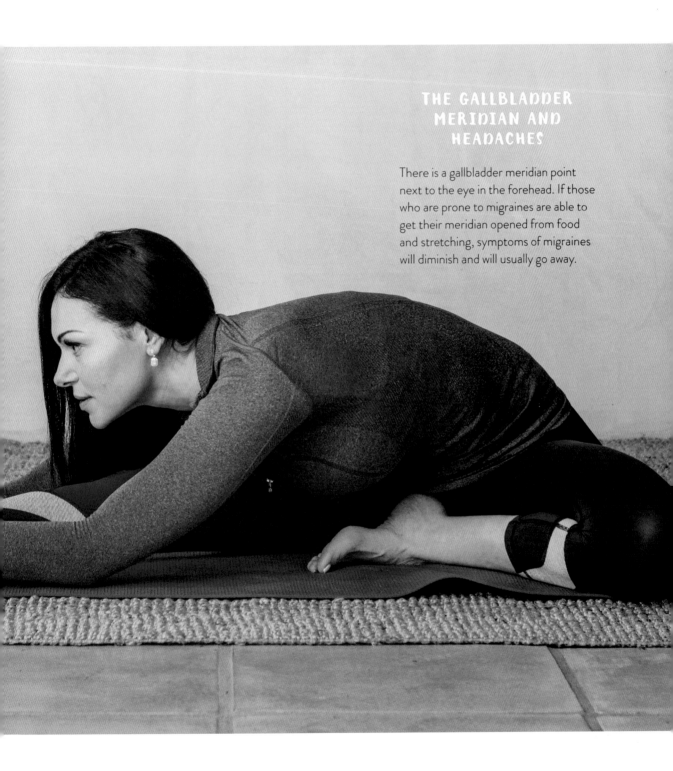

THE GALLBLADDER MERIDIAN AND HEADACHES

There is a gallbladder meridian point next to the eye in the forehead. If those who are prone to migraines are able to get their meridian opened from food and stretching, symptoms of migraines will diminish and will usually go away.

Psychological Traits of Your Gallbladder and Liver

In Chinese Meridian Theory, different organs are affiliated with different psychological traits. When you eat the right way and stretch properly, these meridians are opened and flow smoothly, allowing what's called the "high sides" to flourish. When the meridians are blocked, however, the "low sides" tend to be exhibited. As you follow the Stash Plan, you will find that the high-side traits will raise and the low-side traits will diminish.

GALLBLADDER HIGH-SIDE TRAITS

- Certainty
- Courageousness
- Decisiveness
- Dependability
- Loyalty

GALLBLADDER LOW-SIDE TRAITS

- Cowardice
- Demeaning of your abilities
- Dependency on people or substances
- Guilty about things
- Indecisiveness

LIVER HIGH-SIDE TRAITS

- Freedom
- Helpfulness
- Independence
- Pride
- Unrepressed

LIVER LOW-SIDE TRAITS

- Being in denial
- Codependence
- Feeling you can't change your life
- Frustration
- Irritability

THE WORST FOODS FOR FASCIA

Junk food or anything processed that your body doesn't recognize as pure untainted food wreaks havoc on your fascia. Particularly harmful are all GMOs, soy, high-fructose corn syrup, refined sugars, and complex white carbohydrates. When you eat too much of this kind of food, it has to be stored somewhere, which is why it usually ends up getting dumped in places where you don't want it, such as your butt and upper thighs.

Stretching and Your Fascia

THE STASH PLAN STRETCHES target your fascia, a highly complex and extremely understudied organ, in a unique way. As we touched on in earlier chapters, fascia is defined as a sheet or band of fibrous connective tissue enveloping, separating, surrounding, or binding together muscles, organs, and other soft structures of the body to hold them in place. This includes the brain, spinal cord, nerves, and abdominal cavity. Recent research, in fact, defines fascia as *all* collagenous material in the body, including ligaments and tendons. This is also why improving your collagen levels with your daily broth is such an important part of our program.

Fascia helps our organs function better, through movement and energy. But if the fascia is too constricted, it can hinder the organ's functioning, as well as cause cellulite.

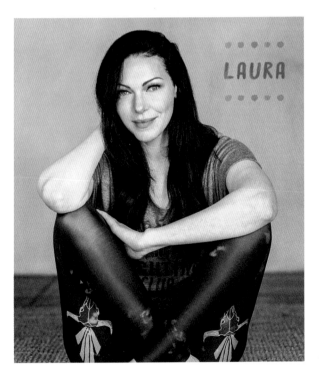

LAURA

When I first started stretching with Elizabeth, I really got perspective on what changes I needed in my body. For the first time, I felt I was finally working with someone who really understood the true anatomy and energy of how the body works. I didn't want to be sick and numb anymore. M3 started to wake me up. I started to actually *feel* my body and get the body I always wanted. Instead of all of the pounding I had done with my crazy workouts, I got longer, leaner, more graceful, and more comfortable in my skin. Firing up my gallbladder and liver meridians opened the floodgates to where my body could actually go. Doing my Stash stretches every day not only keeps me on target but gives me the confidence to know that I'm doing the very best I can for my muscles and my overall health.

ELIZABETH

A discovery I made while developing M3, based on Chinese Meridian Theory, was being able to link organs to a specific body part or muscle group. I found that if its meridian is stretched and fired, the organ functions better. An interesting point: Tendons are linked to the liver and ligaments are linked to the gallbladder—they rely on the nourishment of the blood filtered from the liver. Movements of limbs and joints are the result of tendons flexing and ligaments extending. The liver stores blood; the heart circulates blood. When the body moves, blood circulates in its channels. When the body is at rest, the blood flows back to the liver for storage. Therefore, if the liver's blood is stagnant and the body is not in motion, the tendons and ligaments become tight and impair agility. Stash stretching is the key to opening everything up again, and when you follow the Stash Plan, this is precisely what happens:

- The targeted stretching fires these meridians so that the organs function better. It pulls the fascia away from the muscle with your own strength, making it possible for meridians to run through them efficiently.

- The broth contains collagen and cartilage to provide deep nourishment for your ligaments and tendons. It also helps heal the gut with easily assimilated micronutrients.

- Real, untainted food improves the overall functioning of the gallbladder and liver while naturally detoxing and nourishing you—and does so without creating the kind of gnarled and knotted-up new fascia caused by eating a chronically unhealthy diet.

HOW TO DO THE
M3 Stretches

THE MOST COMMON BELIEF is that stretching occurs when you elongate muscles, but the secret of Stash stretching is *resistance*.

Think of arm wrestling. Imagine Sylvester Stallone in all his 1980s glory in the movie *Over the Top*. In an arm wrestle, your elbow goes onto the table, your hand clasps your opponent's, and then you resist against this opponent's force in the form of your opponent's arm pressing back—or opposing—yours. This very same concept is at the heart of Stash stretching. Simply, you apply your own force against the opposing muscle group of your own body. Using this force, you pull fascia from the muscle, open up energy pathways, and shoot energy into the gallbladder and liver meridians. This improves the functioning of those organs.

Overflexible and floppy with no muscle tone is not what you want. Nor do you want that super-tight, super-bulky body of someone who practically lives in the weight room at the gym. Resistance creates *true* strength. You get leaner and stronger, and you can easily become so in only minutes a day.

Many people think it's the muscles that come first, *then* the food, and before now, most didn't think about their meridians. We believe it's the food that comes first, which has a positive effect on the meridian and in turn has a positive effect on muscle and organ function. Conversely, bad food affects the meridian, which jams up the energy, which then stops the muscle and organ from working properly. The good news is that for the first time ever, the Stash Plan teaches you how to address all these facets of food, energy, and your body!

In Part Five, you'll find the basic Muscle Meridian Method stretches to open up and unleash the energy in your gallbladder and liver—allowing for optimum function, energy flow, and fat-burning.

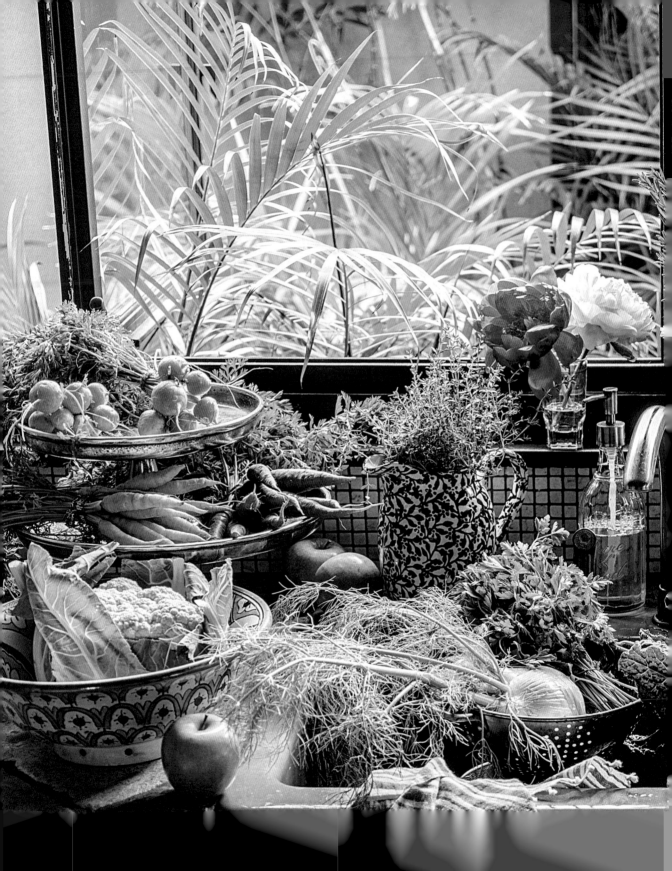

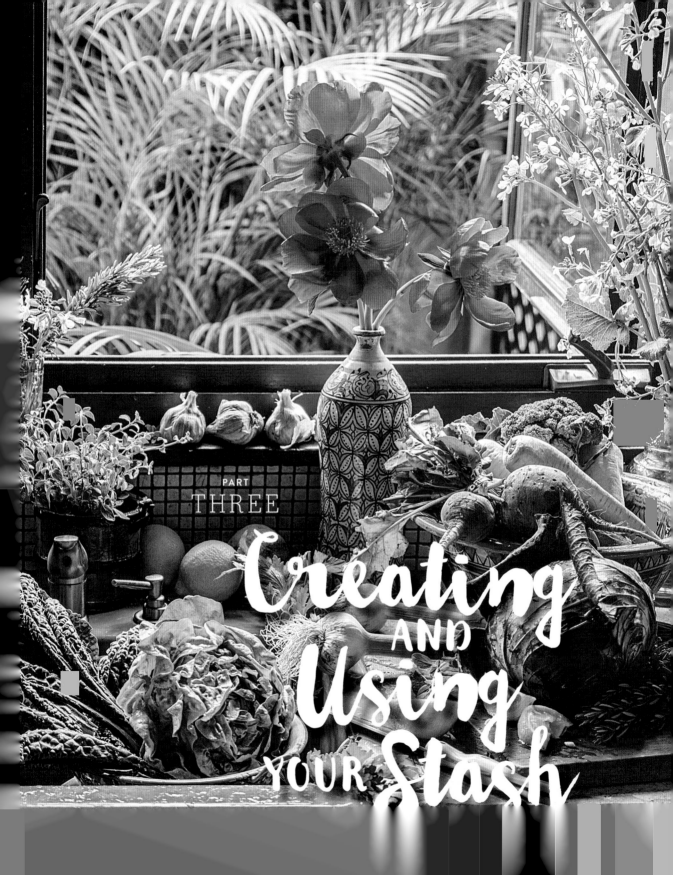

PART
THREE

Creating
AND
Using
YOUR Stash

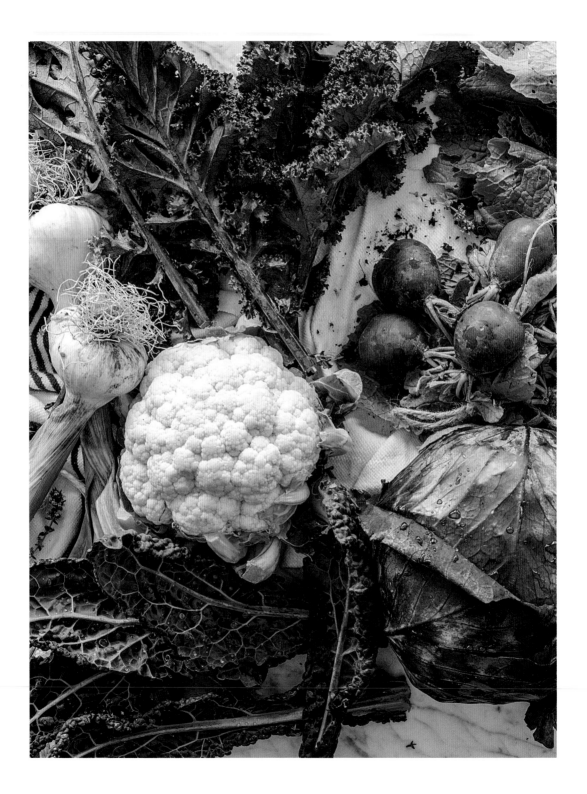

HAVE YOU FOUND YOURSELF

reading a *recipe* or watching a cooking show and
wondering why it looks so easy when you find cooking
so *daunting*? Well, fear not. *Chapter 8* is going to
show you just how **simple** it is to cook the delicious food
you'll be making for your stashes. And then *Chapter 9*
will take you through the fundamentals of Stash building.
You'll soon be a *Stashing pro.*

Kitchen CONFIDENCE

Did you see the Disney movie Ratatouille?
One of the most indelible phrases in it
was "Anyone can cook"—because anyone can!
If you can boil water, turn on an oven, or
slice up some veggies, you can cook.

My confidence in cooking came after I opened my first studio. Many of my clients would come to my seven p.m. class straight from work. I've always had a tendency to make a lot of food, maybe because I am the youngest of five children, three of whom are guys, so large quantities of food at the dinner table were an everyday occurrence. So I would always race home during a few hours of breaks between classes in my studio to make dinner for my family of three. I particularly love soup, and making different ones became my specialty. Because it's impractical to make only a small amount of soup at a time, I'd leave enough for us at home, and bring the enormous pot of soup to my studio for all of my clients to enjoy before, during, and after class. My students began to beg me to give cooking and food education classes, which is why I started teaching food workshops. I spent countless hours researching the effects of specific foods on individual organs, particularly the gallbladder and liver, so I could create recipes and teach about cooking foods with maximum nutritional punch.

Think you don't have time to cook at home? Well, we'll show you how time-effective the cooking process for your weekly Stash can truly be. Once you get your routine established, you won't believe how much more time you'll have, and your weekly Stash parties will bring your family and friends together for lots of fun and healthy eating, or cooking your Stash alone, providing some Zen time in the kitchen, as Laura likes.

Cooking Really Is Easy

Organize Your Food Shopping

- **Start with a list.** We always make shopping lists and organize them by categories so we can find everything we need as quickly and expeditiously as possible. So put all your veggies on one part of the list, your staples on another, your proteins on another, and so on. In most grocery stores, the fresh foods are along the outer aisles and the packaged foods are in the middle, so you'll mostly be sticking to the outside.

- **Never go food shopping when you are really hungry.** It's nearly impossible to not make impulse purchases.

LAURA

I know that people can have a busy day when it's time to Stash Up, but our recipes are so simple to make that you really will be surprised how little time they take. The Stash Plan takes the confusion and complexity out of cooking. Whether you're home or on the go all day, having a Stash means your meals are already taken care of. No more wondering and worrying about what to eat!

Many people, including Elizabeth and me, have endlessly fraught schedules. But we look forward to our weekly Stash time, because not only is it incredibly productive and nourishing, but it becomes a cherished and welcome break from our usual hectic activities. We make two kinds of vegetables, two kinds of protein, and two starch/good carbohydrates. This has been very successful in helping us and others stick to the plan when we know our days are going to be crazy busy.

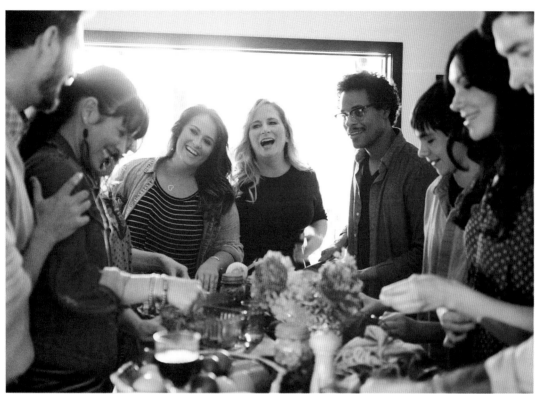

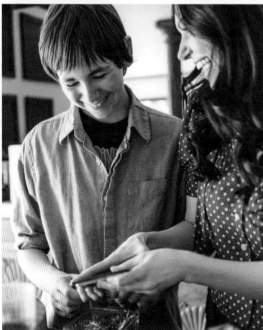

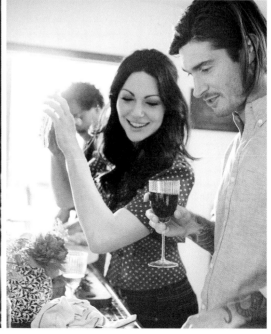

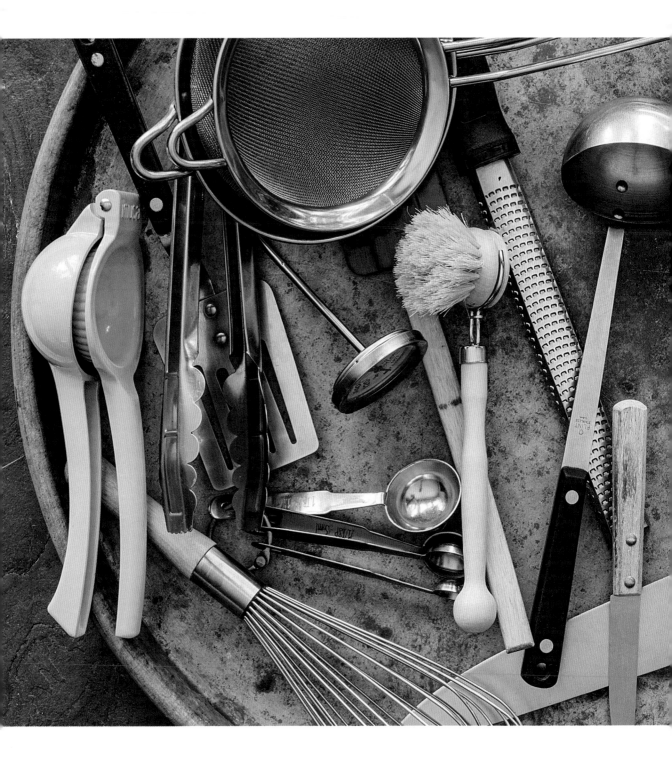

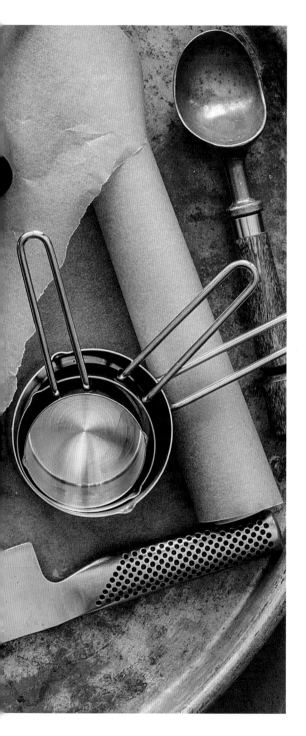

Start Small

Once you master a basic recipe, your confidence will build. Anyone can fill a pot with water, cut up some veggies, throw in a few bones, and add some herbs for flavor. It is deeply satisfying to turn on a slow cooker in the morning and come home at night to a home filled with the mouthwatering aroma of a super-nutritious food that basically cooked itself!

Cooking Is Therapeutic—and Fun!

One of the things we love most about Stashing is that it brings us close to our food. We choose it, touch it, examine it, cut it up, transform it, and then eat it. Hands-on cooking helps you connect to the beauty, energy, texture, and aroma of the food you eat. Smelling good food is good for the soul; seeing and tasting it is even better.

What a pleasure it is to eat good food!

• • • • ELIZABETH • • • •

I think one of the biggest mistakes anyone can make when cooking is taking it too seriously. You need to have fun and be willing to make mistakes. When Laura and I first sat down to start our original outline for our Stash Plan, we both felt our priority was to help people, to educate them—and for our readers to have fun! The concepts in the Stash Plan are so simple, yet the impact on our lives is so huge! I always tell my clients that my favorite tips are to relax with cooking, to experiment and try new things, and to always create time to build their Stashes. The investment is worth it!

ESSENTIAL EQUIPMENT

APPLIANCES AND EQUIPMENT

- Aluminum foil
- Blender (*Laura: I love my Vitamix blender. It is incredibly powerful and can chop, puree, and liquefy; it's great for making soups.*)
- Cheesecloth
- Cooking twine
- Cutting board
- Fat separator (good to use for drinking a cup of broth before refrigerating it)
- Food processor
- Grater
- Lemon juicer
- Potholders
- Slow cooker
- Strainers, one small handheld and one large metal freestanding
- Toaster
- Toaster oven (optional)
- Waxed paper bags and roll, unbleached
- Wire rack

POTS AND PANS

- Cookie sheets
- Dutch oven
- Large nonstick skillet, with cover
- Small nonstick loaf pan for bread and meat loaf
- Roasting pans, small, medium, and large
- Roasting rack
- Saucepans, small, medium, and large, with lids
- Skillets, small, medium, and large, with lids
- Stockpot

UTENSILS

- Heatproof stirring spoons
- Kitchen shears
- Knives
- Ladle
- Large fork
- Measuring cups and spoons
- Parer
- Rubber or silicone food scraper
- Tongs
- Vegetable chopper (optional) (*Laura: I love my vegetable chopper. I first got one after my friend sold them in a mall and gave me one as a present. He had a whole sales pitch when selling them and gave chopping demos. It was very funny. One thing I always remembered from his pitch was "no more tears!" So for cutting onions, I love to use my vegetable chopper because it really helps with the crying factor. I also love it for mincing garlic and herbs.*)
- Vegetable scrubber (*optional, but it makes cleaning the veggies a lot easier, especially if you aren't peeling them*)
- Whisk

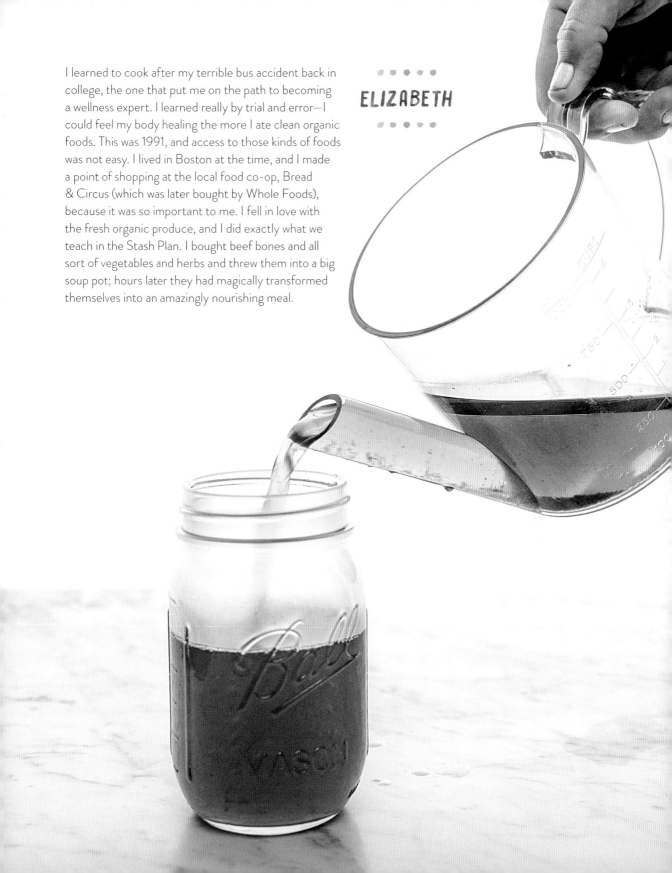

I learned to cook after my terrible bus accident back in college, the one that put me on the path to becoming a wellness expert. I learned really by trial and error—I could feel my body healing the more I ate clean organic foods. This was 1991, and access to those kinds of foods was not easy. I lived in Boston at the time, and I made a point of shopping at the local food co-op, Bread & Circus (which was later bought by Whole Foods), because it was so important to me. I fell in love with the fresh organic produce, and I did exactly what we teach in the Stash Plan. I bought beef bones and all sort of vegetables and herbs and threw them into a big soup pot; hours later they had magically transformed themselves into an amazingly nourishing meal.

ELIZABETH

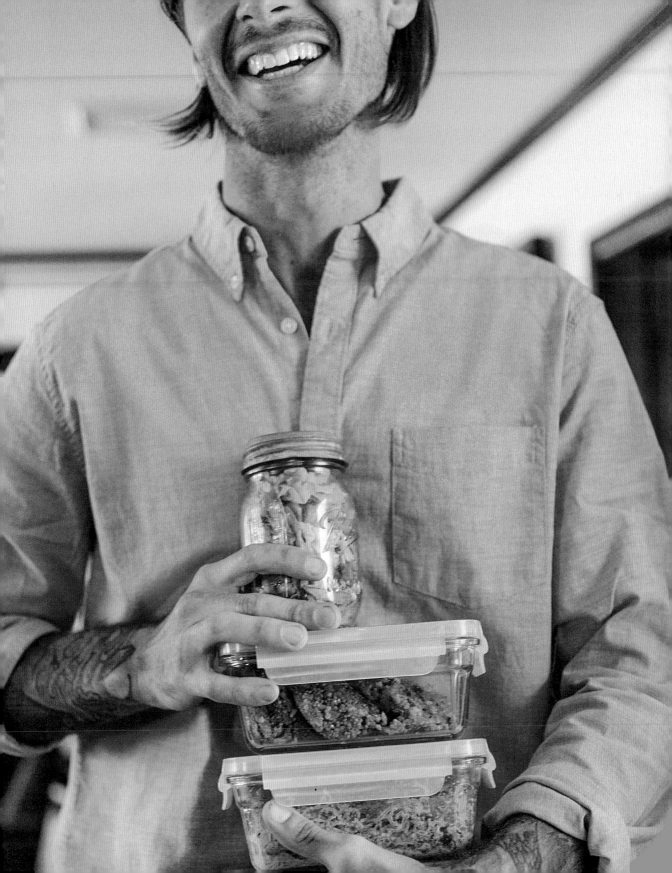

STASH CONTAINERS—
HOW TO STASH YOUR STASH

LAURA The best containers to use for your stash are glass.
Be aware that if you use plastic, there is a very high risk for the
PCBs (polychlorinated biphenyl) found in plastics to leach into
the food, especially if heated in a microwave—which is a habit
everyone should break—or if left in the sun (as can happen
with bottled water). PCBs have been demonstrated to cause
cancer and to have a variety of other adverse health effects on
the immune system, reproductive system, nervous system, and
endocrine system. It is not a risk worth taking for the conve-
nience of using lightweight, unbreakable Tupperware or other
plastic containers, even if marked "microwave-safe"! To make
your delicious, nutritious Stash and then put it in plastic totally
defeats the purpose.

When I go to the set, I have a special backpack designated
to carry my Stash. You can easily find sets of nesting glass
containers with tight-fitting lids online, and you can use a large
thermos for your broth or heat it up at work. My castmates and
crew always want to know what I'm going to be bringing every
day, and slowly, more and more people are starting to bring their
own food to set.

chapter 9

Stash

BUILDING,

MEAL PLANS, AND

STASH

1

*So here we are, ready to finally get to the good
stuff—how to prepare the food! You now
know all the best foods to eat, and you're going
to see how to create the first of six sample Stashes
in this book. And once the basic ingredients
are prepared, you'll learn how to incorporate it
all into delicious, filling meals.*

A quick reminder: You'll do all your cooking on the two Stash-up days each week. Then pop all the food in the fridge. Each morning you assemble the meals for the day using the precooked food, making healthy eating and sticking to the Stash Plan effortless. This chapter will give you the in-depth directions for how to prepare Stash 1. You can then find Stashes 2 through 6 in Chapter 11, waiting for you to become a Stashing machine!

How to Build a Stash

NOW THAT YOU KNOW which foods will unstick and help heal your gallbladder and liver, it's time to maximize their potential and put them all together for your stashes. Here's what to do:

- Twice a week you will be making your Stash food, and then you'll be able to prepare meals from this for the next three days and create a stronger sense of connection to the foods that will be healing you. We will also give you tips and shortcuts that will cut down on preparation time.

- Each week you will have two Stash-up days. On Stash-up Day One, you will make foods for Monday through Wednesday. On Stash-up Day Two, you will make your Stash for Thursday through Saturday. Sunday is a day off—we are 80/20, after all!—but you will still have your broth and make sure you are eating GMO-free, organic food whenever possible.

- The Stashes include two proteins, two vegetable sides, two grains, hand grabbers (quick snacks), and a broth. Each day's meals will be combinations of these yummy parts.

- Your Stash building for the day should take no more than ten minutes. You just assemble and divide your meals into portable glass containers, and you're done!

- These Stashes are enough for four days of meals. These foods are specifically geared toward unblocking your gallbladder and liver, and are packed with antioxidants.

LAURA

I usually pack up my Stash meals cold and then heat them when I get to set. However, some recipes are meant to be room temperature, and most of the recipes taste great at room temperature regardless! Filming in New York City in the colder months, I found it nice to have a hot meal, so what's great about the Stash Plan is that you can tweak it however it works best for you. I also usually heat my broth in the morning and pack it in a thermos, so it's hot all day for me to enjoy whenever I want. You might like to do the same.

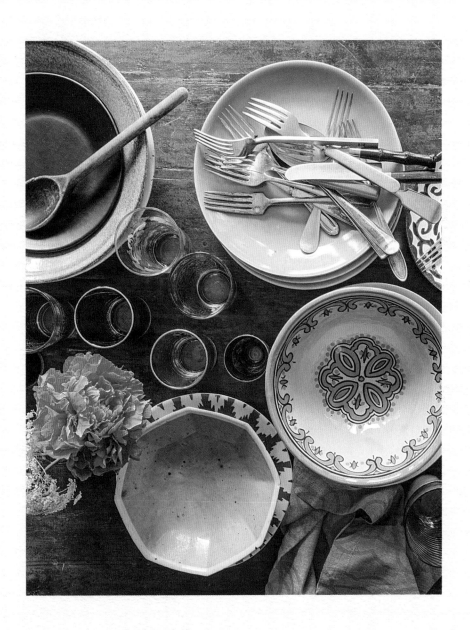

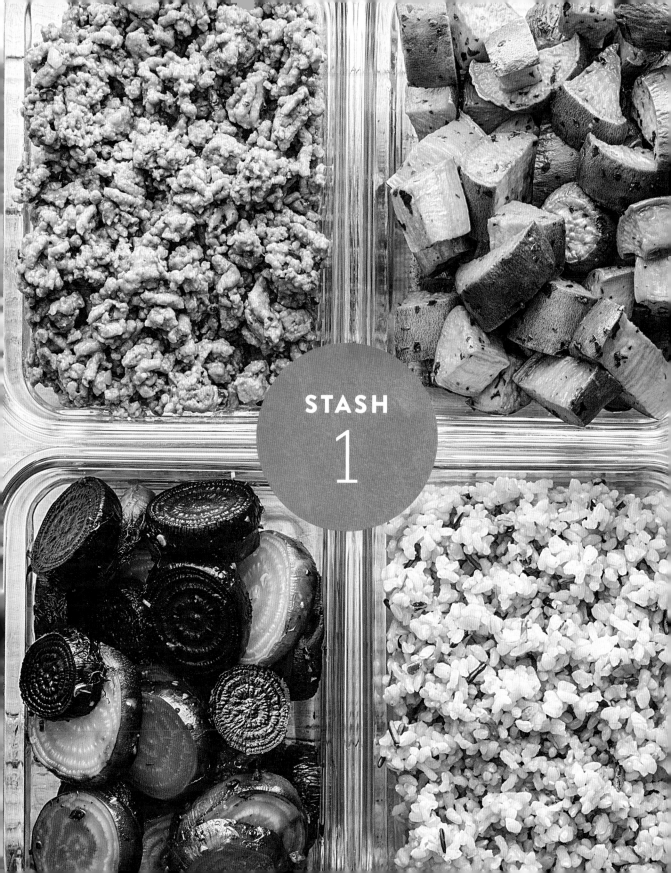

STASH

1

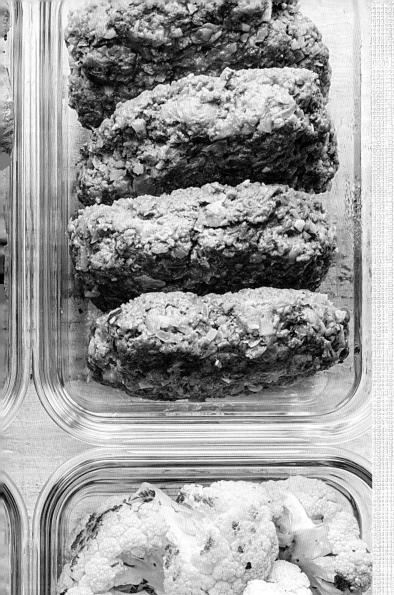

BROTH

- Basic Beef Broth (page 195)

PROTEIN

- "No Bull" Bison Patties
- Turmeric Turkey

CARBS

- Herb-Roasted Sweet Potato Home Fries
- Broth-Infused Brown Rice

VEGGIES

- Garlic-Roasted Beets
- Roasted Cauliflower

HAND GRABBERS

- almond butter
- almonds
- Hass avocado
- blueberries
- butter lettuce
- dried coconut flakes
- eggs
- Gluten-Free Almond Bread
- Granny Smith apples
- spinach
- walnuts

STASH 1: SHOPPING LIST

NOTE: *As you will see below, because this is the first Stash, you will need to buy some pantry items and hand grabbers. In addition, all food items, including spices, should be organic.*

SAUCES AND CONDIMENTS

- almond butter, 16-ounce jar
- apple cider vinegar, 16-ounce bottle
- Braggs Liquid Amino Acids, 16-ounce bottle
- brown rice syrup, 16-ounce jar
- olive oil, 16-ounce bottle
- pure maple syrup, 12-ounce bottle
- raw honey, 22-ounce jar
- ume plum vinegar, 5-ounce bottle

HERBS AND SPICES
(All herbs and spices should be bought by spice container)

- bay leaves
- black peppercorns, in a grinder
- black peppercorns, whole
- cayenne pepper
- cinnamon
- cloves
- cumin
- dried oregano
- garlic powder
- Himalayan pink salt
- mustard seeds
- paprika
- Real Salt (sea salt)
- turmeric, ground

FLOUR AND GRAINS

- almond flour, 12-ounce bag
- baking soda, 1 pound box
- coconut flour, 16-ounce bag
- quinoa, 16-ounce bag
- quinoa noodles, 1 box
- millet, 16-ounce box
- purple rice, 16-ounce bag
- short grain brown rice, 16-ounce bag

NUTS, SEEDS, AND FLAKES

- almonds, 1 cup (about 5 ounces)
- coconut flakes, dried unsweetened, 16-ounce bag
- flaxseeds, ground, 12-ounce bag
- pine nuts, 8-ounce bag
- sunflower seeds, 16-ounce bag
- walnuts, 16-ounce bag

FOOD FOR RECIPES

- 1 pound grass-fed bone marrow
- 1 pound grass-fed knuckle bones
- 1 pound grass-fed bone-in short ribs
- 1 pound ground bison meat
- 1 pound hormone-free ground turkey meat (white and dark)
- 7 large beets (yellow and red)
- 1½ pound bag of carrots
- 2 heads of cauliflower

- 1 pound bunch of celery
- 1 bunch of cilantro
- 1 large bunch of flat-leaf Italian parsley
- 1 large fresh piece of ginger
- 2 heads of garlic
- 1 bunch of fresh mint
- 2 large yellow onions
- 1 bunch of rosemary
- 1 bunch of thyme
- 2 large sweet potatoes
- 1 pound butter
- 1 large container of yogurt
- 1 Hass avocado
- 1 container of blueberries
- 1 butter lettuce
- 1 dozen eggs
- 3 Granny Smith apples
- 1 bag of spinach

AND OUT OF THIS SHOPPING LIST, HERE'S WHAT YOU SHOULD HAVE LEFT OVER FOR USE IN YOUR WEEK 2 STASH

- approximately 6 to 8 carrots
- approximately 6 to 8 stalks of celery
- ginger
- approximately 6 tablespoons of mint
- ¾ bunch of rosemary
- ¾ bunch of thyme
- butter
- 1 cup spinach
- 3 eggs

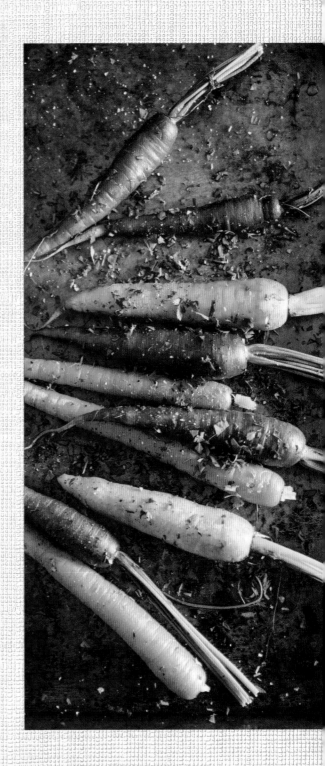

STASH 1: COOK AND PREPARE

1. THE NIGHT BEFORE

Prepare Your Rice

(This should take less than 10 minutes.)

- Place 1 cup brown rice in a bowl.
- Add ¼ cup wild rice (optional).
- Add 3 tablespoons Greek yogurt.
- Pour on 1½ cups water.
- Stir until yogurt dissolves.
- Leave on counter overnight to ferment.

Prepare Your Broth

When you chop the vegetables, they don't have to be pretty—the more rustic, the better!

- Place 1 pound marrowbones and 1 pound knucklebones in slow cooker.
- Add two carrots chopped in big chunks.
- Add 2 celery stalks chopped in big chunks.

- Add one full head garlic (chop off the top portion; do not worry about peeling it).
- Add one whole onion cut in half (do not worry about peeling it).
- Add a 2-inch piece of fresh ginger (do not worry about peeling it).
- Add 2 sprigs rosemary.
- Add 2 sprigs thyme.
- Add 2 teaspoons Real Salt (or sea salt of your choice).
- Add 2 teaspoons whole black peppercorns.
- Add water to 2 inches above the ingredients. Cook on high in slow cooker for at least 15 hours. You want a slow simmer.

••• LAURA •••

I like to cook my broth on high for about 15 to 20 hours in a slow cooker. I also give it a few stirs during the cooking process and poke the marrow out of the marrowbones with a knife once it's been cooking for several hours, and then stir. Every slow cooker or stove is different. You want the broth to be on a low simmer, with bubbles every few seconds.

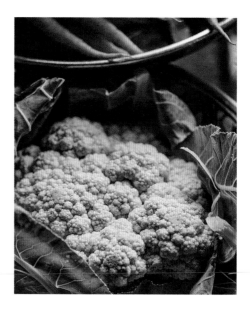

2. COOK YOUR STASH

More detailed recipes are in the next section.

- Preheat oven to 350°F.
- Place 6 bowls on the counter.
- Rinse and dry beets, sweet potatoes, cauliflower, and herbs.
- Chop 2 large sweet potatoes and place in a bowl.
- Chop two heads of cauliflower and place in a bowl.
- Cut the ends off the beets, pare off the skin (doesn't have to be perfect), then cut into chunks and put into a bowl. (Red beets will make your hands red, so you can wear rubber gloves while doing this or rinse your hands afterward.)
- Discard parings and wipe down cutting board with a damp cloth, so the red from the beets doesn't get on the other food.
- Chop 1 onion with chopper (optional) or knife and place in a bowl.
- Chop 4 cloves of garlic with chopper or knife and place in a bowl.
- Chop one head of cilantro with chopper or knife.
- Chop parsley (2 tablespoons) with chopper or knife.
- Chop mint (1 tablespoon) with chopper or knife.

- Place 3 baking sheets on the counter. Cover one with beets, one with sweet potatoes, and one with cauliflower. Drizzle 1¼ tablespoons of olive oil over each pan.
- Sprinkle sweet potatoes with 1 tablespoon parsley (save the rest for the bison patties).
- Sprinkle cauliflower with 2 tablespoons cilantro.
- Sprinkle beets with 1 tablespoon garlic.
- Sprinkle each baking sheet with 1 teaspoon salt and 1 teaspoon pepper. Massage ingredients into the veggies. Place all three baking sheets into the oven, set timer for 15 minutes.
- Place one medium skillet on the stove, with 1 tablespoon olive oil over medium-low heat. Add onions and garlic. Cook onions until they are translucent , about 5–8 minutes.
- Wipe out the large bowl the cauliflower was in and place bison meat inside.
- At this point the 15-minute timer will go off. Stir veggies to help them cook evenly. Set timer for another 5 minutes.
- Back to bison meat. Add sautéed onion and garlic mixture to the bison in the bowl.
- Add the rest of the parsley, mint, ½ teaspoon salt, and ½ teaspoon pepper. Mix all together with your hands.

(continues)

- Shape bison meat into 4 equal-sized oval patties.

- Timer goes off around now. Take cauliflower out of the oven, leave on counter to cool.

- Set timer for 10 minutes.

- Back to bison meat. Place 1 large skillet on the stove and heat on low heat with 2 teaspoons of olive oil. Place patties in the pan. Add 1 tablespoon broth and cook for 5 minutes on low heat.

- Around now the oven timer goes off. Pull beets out and leave on counter to cool. Set timer for 10 more minutes.

- Back to bison. Flip patties, add 1 tablespoon broth. Cover bison and cook for 3–4 minutes on medium low. Then, transfer to a glass storage container; allow to cool.

- Around now the timer should go off. Take out sweet potatoes and leave on counter to cool.

- Set oven heat to 325°F.

- Rinse out bison skillet and place back on the stove. Heat over medium heat with 1 tablespoon olive oil. Place ground turkey in the skillet. Add ¼ cup broth, leftover cilantro, ¼ teaspoon cayenne, ½ teaspoon salt, ½ teaspoon pepper, 1½ teaspoons turmeric, ¼ teaspoon cumin.

- Break up turkey with a spatula while it cooks. Add an additional ¼ cup broth.

Cook for a total of 8–10 minutes, stirring frequently to avoid overcooking. Place in a glass container, allow to cool.

- Rinse rice and place in a pot over medium heat. Add ½ cup broth, 1½ cups water, and 1 teaspoon salt. Bring to a boil, then reduce heat to low and cover.

- Grease your small loaf pan.

- In a food processor, combine 2 cups almond flour, 2 tablespoons coconut flour, ¼ cup ground flaxseeds, ½ teaspoon baking soda, and ½ teaspoon sea salt. Add 5 large eggs, 1½ tablespoons honey, 1 tablespoon olive oil, and 1 tablespoon apple cider vinegar. Pulse about 5 times to blend. Pour mixture into the loaf pan. Place in the 325° oven and cook for 20 minutes.

- Back to rice. It should be finished now; transfer to a glass container and allow to cool.

- Back to almond bread. Cover with foil and return to the oven for another 10 minutes, or until a toothpick comes out clean from the middle. Let it cool for about 20 minutes.

- Place veggies in covered glass containers and transfer to the fridge. Wrap bread or place in a glass container.

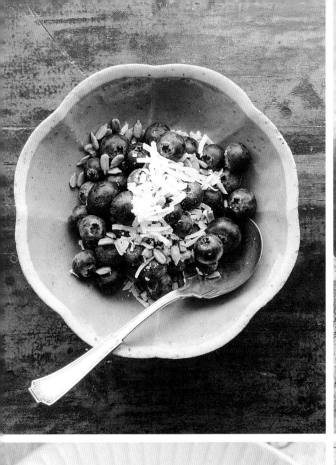

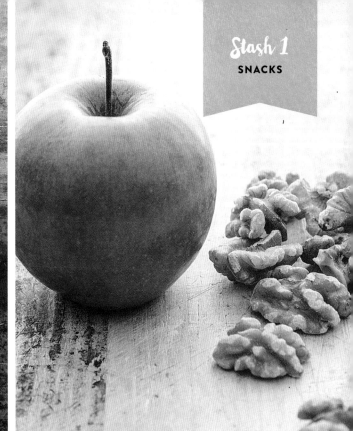

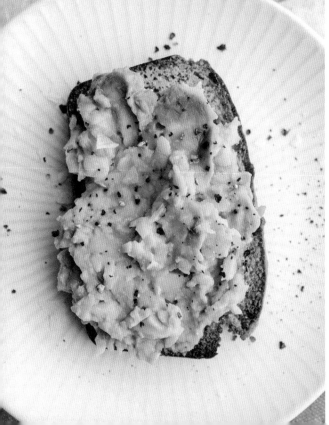

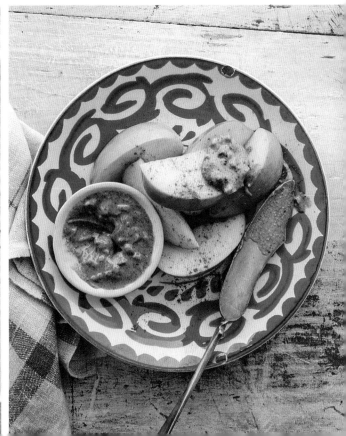

Monday

MEAL 1

- 4 ounces Turmeric Turkey
- 1 cup Roasted Cauliflower
- ½ cup Broth-Infused Brown Rice

Snack

- 1 Granny Smith apple
- 10 walnuts

MEAL 2

- 1 "No Bull" Bison Patty
- 1 cup Garlic-Roasted Beets
- ½ cup Broth-Infused Brown Rice
- 2 cups butter lettuce
- Slice patty. Wrap in butter lettuce.

Snack

- Avocado Toast

  Toast 1 slice of Gluten-Free Almond Bread. Smash ½ avocado on top. Add salt and pepper to taste.

MEAL 3

- 4 ounces Turmeric Turkey
- 1 cup Garlic-Roasted Beets
- ½ cup of Herb-Roasted Sweet Potato Home Fries

Tuesday

MEAL 1

- 2 eggs, fried
- ½ cup Broth-Infused Brown Rice
- 1 cup Roasted Cauliflower

Snack

- 1 Granny Smith apple, sliced and sprinkled with cinnamon, if desired
- 2 tablespoons almond butter

MEAL 2

- 4 ounces Turmeric Turkey
- 1 cup Garlic-Roasted Beets
- 2 slices Avocado Toast
- ½ Hass avocado

  Toast 2 slices of Gluten-Free Almond Bread. Smash ½ avocado on top. Place half of the turkey on each slice and gently press down so it sticks to the avocado. Add salt and pepper to taste. Top with butter lettuce.

Snack

- 1 cup blueberries
- 2 tablespoons sunflower seeds
- 1 tablespoon coconut flakes

MEAL 3

- 1 "No Bull" Bison Patty
- ½ cup Broth-Infused Brown Rice
- 1 cup Garlic-Roasted Beets

Wednesday

MEAL 1

- 2 eggs, scrambled in 1 tablespoon of butter with 1 cup chopped spinach
- ½ cup Broth-Infused Brown Rice

Snack

- Avocado Toast

  Toast 1 slice of Gluten-Free Almond Bread. Smash ½ avocado on top. Add salt and pepper to taste.

MEAL 2

- 1 "No Bull" Bison Patty
- 1 cup Roasted Cauliflower
- ½ cup Herb-Roasted Sweet Potato Home Fries

Snack

- 1 Granny Smith apple, sliced and sprinkled with cinnamon, if desired

MEAL 3

- 4 ounces Turmeric Turkey
- 1 cup Garlic-Roasted Beets
- ½ cup Broth-Infused Brown Rice

  Place turkey and beets over a bed of spinach and butter lettuce drizzled with 1 tablespoon olive oil.

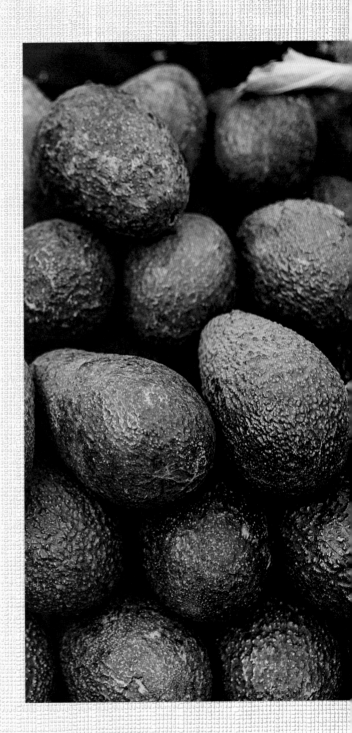

BROTH-INFUSED
BROWN RICE

ROASTED
CAULIFLOWER

TURMERIC TURKEY

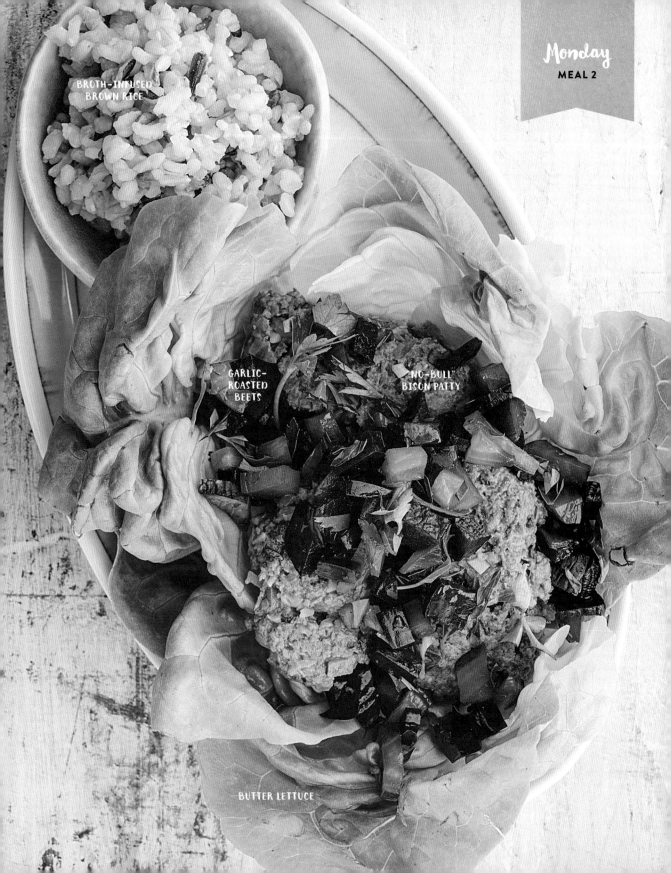

BROTH-INFUSED
BROWN RICE

GARLIC-
ROASTED
BEETS

"NO-BULL"
BISON PATTY

BUTTER LETTUCE

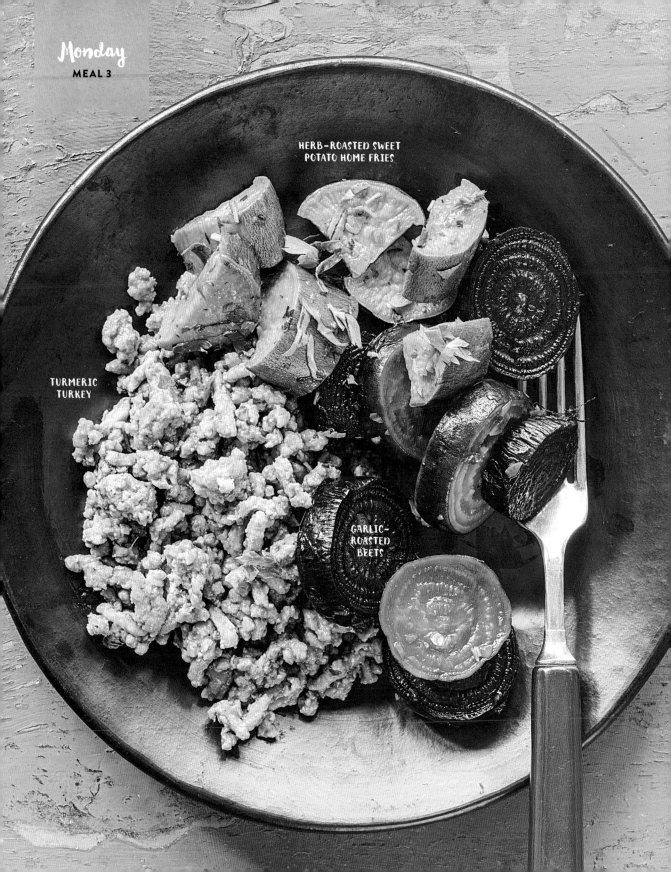

HERB-ROASTED SWEET
POTATO HOME FRIES

TURMERIC
TURKEY

GARLIC-
ROASTED
BEETS

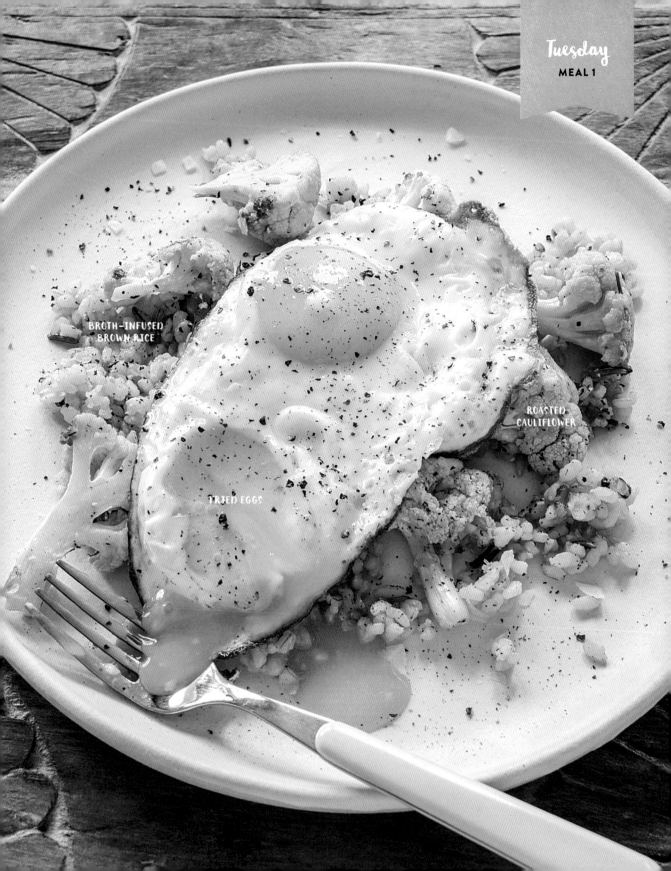

Tuesday
MEAL 1

BROTH-INFUSED
BROWN RICE

ROASTED
CAULIFLOWER

FRIED EGGS

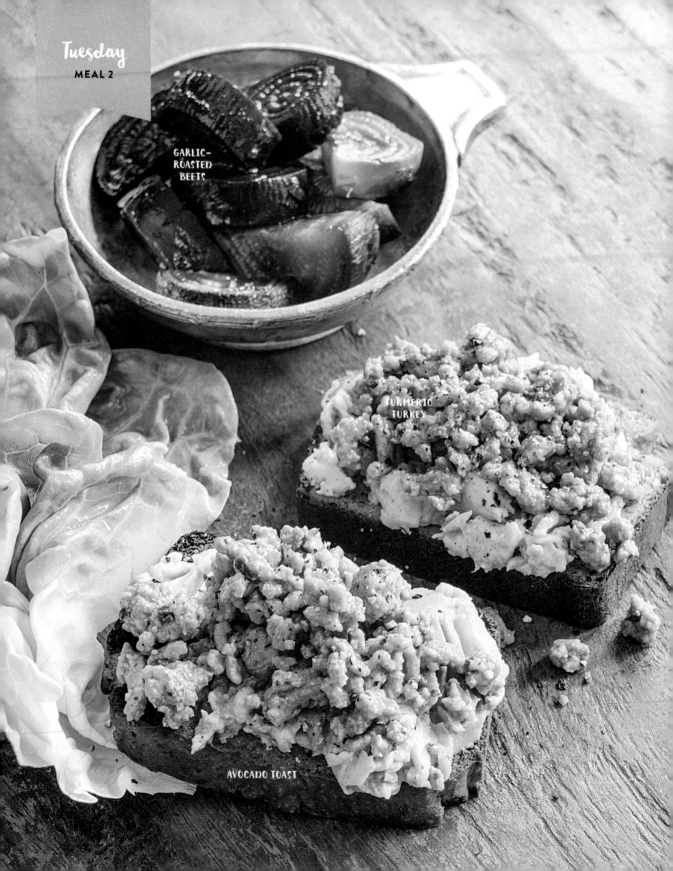

GARLIC-
ROASTED
BEETS

TURMERIC
TURKEY

AVOCADO TOAST

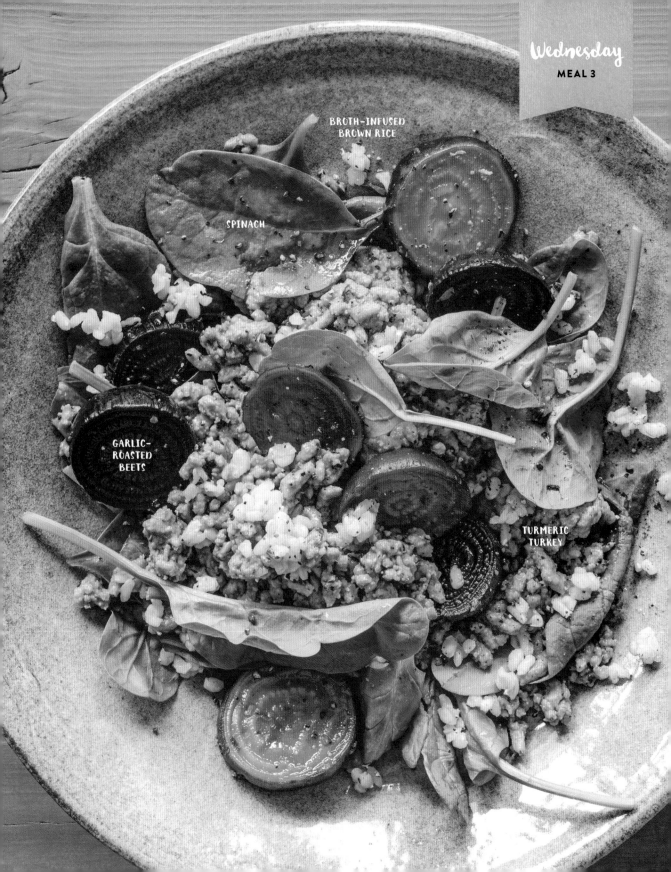

BROTH-INFUSED
BROWN RICE

SPINACH

GARLIC-
ROASTED
BEETS

TURMERIC
TURKEY

STASH 1
PROTEIN

"no bull" bison patties

2 tablespoons olive oil
1 large yellow onion, chopped
3 cloves garlic, minced
1 pound grass-fed ground bison meat
1 tablespoon chopped flat-leaf Italian parsley
1 teaspoon minced fresh mint
½ teaspoon Real Salt
½ teaspoon fresh-ground black pepper
2 tablespoons beef broth (page 195)

1. Heat a skillet over medium heat. Add 1 tablespoon olive oil, onion, and garlic. Cook, stirring occasionally, for 5 minutes until onions are translucent. Remove from heat and allow to cool.

2. Place bison meat into a bowl. Add parsley, onion mixture, mint, salt, and pepper. Shape mixture into 4 oblong patties.

3. Heat a skillet over medium heat with 1 tablespoon olive oil. Place all four patties in the pan with 1 tablespoon of the broth. Cook for 2 minutes, then cover. Cook for another 2 minutes. Flip patties, pour additional 1 tablespoon of broth in the middle of the pan, and cover. Let the patties cook for another 4 minutes.

4. Place patties on a plate and allow to cool.

LAURA

I usually test to see if the patties have finished cooking by pressing on the top of a patty. If it's a firm spring, they are done.

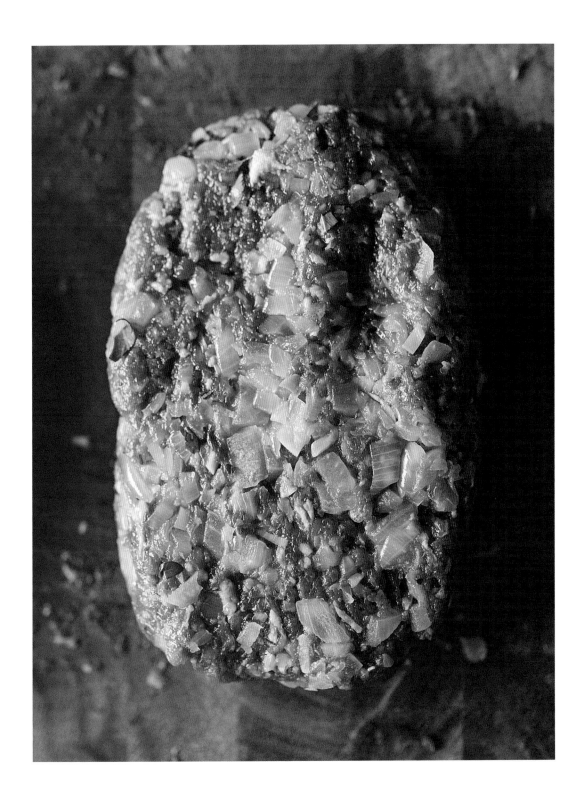

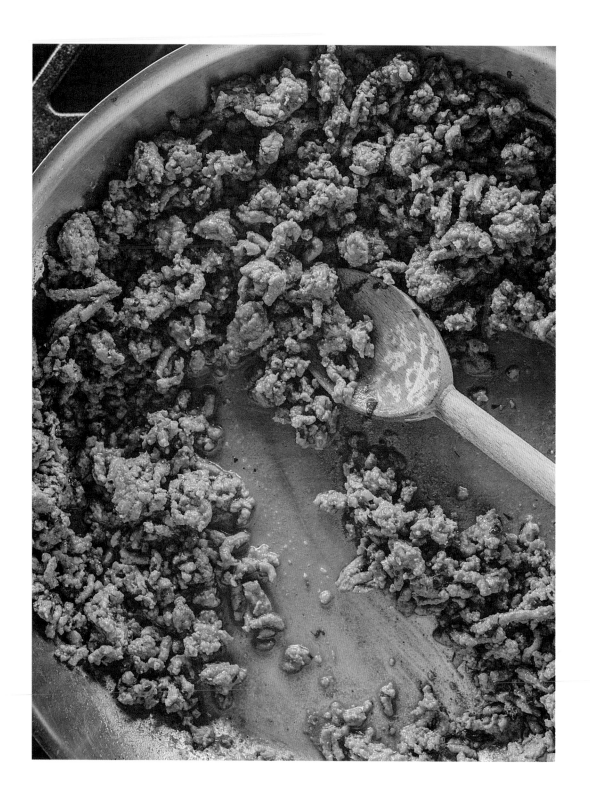

turmeric turkey

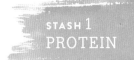

1 tablespoon olive oil

1 pound ground white-meat turkey

½ cup beef broth

2 tablespoons chopped cilantro

½ teaspoon Real Salt

¼ teaspoon fresh-ground black pepper

2 teaspoons turmeric

¼ teaspoon cumin

¼ teaspoon cayenne pepper

1. Heat a skillet over medium heat. Add olive oil and turkey. Break the turkey into chunks with a thick metal spatula.

2. Add ¼ cup broth, cilantro, salt, pepper, turmeric, cumin, and cayenne. Continue to break up the turkey into small pieces as you stir all ingredients together.

3. Cook for 4 minutes. Add remaining ¼ cup beef broth, and cook for another 4 minutes.

4. Allow to cool, then transfer to a glass container.

STASH 1
CARBS

herb-roasted sweet potato home fries

2 large sweet potatoes
1¼ tablespoons olive oil
1 tablespoon minced flat-leaf Italian parsley
1 teaspoon Real Salt
1 teaspoon fresh-ground black pepper
1¼ tablespoons olive oil

1. Preheat oven to 350°F. Rinse and dry sweet potatoes. Cut ends off, then cut into slices an inch thick. Cut these slices into 1- to 2-inch cubes.

2. Place sweet potatoes on a baking sheet. Drizzle with olive oil, then add parsley and salt. Toss with your hands to coat well.

3. Place in the oven and roast for 15 minutes. Stir with a spatula, flipping the sweet potatoes over, then roast for an additional 20 minutes, or until a knife can easily pierce them.

4. Allow to cool, then transfer to a glass container.

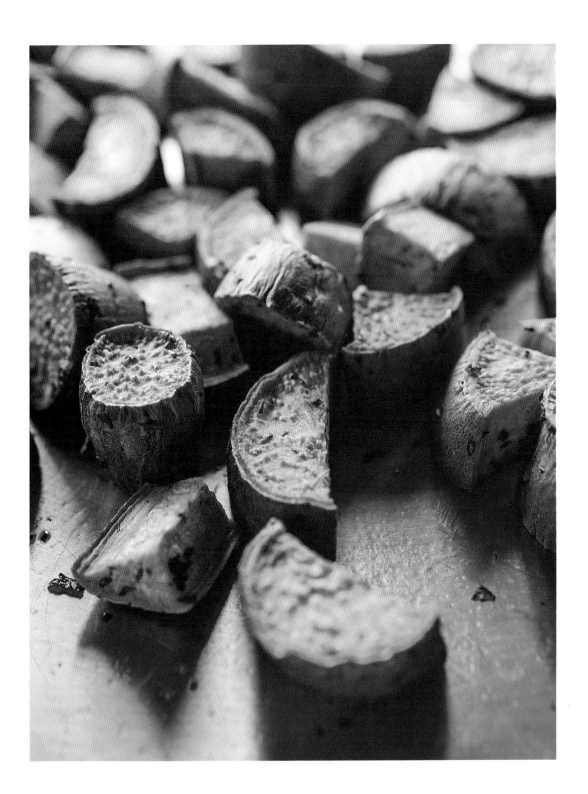

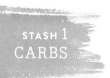

STASH 1
CARBS

broth-infused brown rice

1 cup short-grain brown rice
¼ cup wild rice (optional)
3 tablespoons plain Greek yogurt
3½ cups water
½ cup beef broth
1 teaspoon Real Salt

ELIZABETH

We soak brown rice (as well as other grains) in yogurt because the yogurt has enzymes that predigest the rice, making it easier for the body to assimilate the nutrients. (It adds flavor as well.)

1. The night before, place rice and wild rice in a glass bowl. Add 3 tablespoons yogurt and 1½ cups of water. Mix until the yogurt is dissolved. Leave on the counter overnight. (This ferments the rice so it's easier to digest.)

2. The next day, put the rice in a strainer and rinse until the water runs clear.

3. Place the rice in a 4-quart saucepan. Add broth, 2 cups water, and salt. Cook on high until the rice begins to boil, then lower the flame to low, cover, and cook for 30 minutes, stirring occasionally.

4. Stir, then allow to cool, then transfer to a glass container.

garlic-roasted beets

7 large beets (red and yellow)
1¼ tablespoons olive oil
1 teaspoon minced garlic
1 teaspoon Real Salt

1. Preheat oven to 350°F. Rinse beets with water and dry. Cut off both ends.

2. Pare the beets. (They don't have to be pretty; it's nice to see a little skin left.) Cut beets into large chunks and place on a baking sheet.

3. Drizzle the olive oil over the beets, then add garlic and salt. Toss with your hands to coat well.

4. Place in the oven and roast for 15 minutes. Stir with a spatula, flipping the beets over, then roast for an additional 10 minutes, or until a knife can easily pierce them.

5. Allow to cool, then transfer to a glass container.

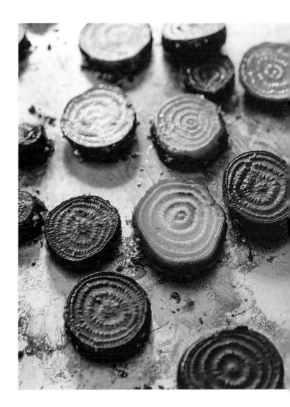

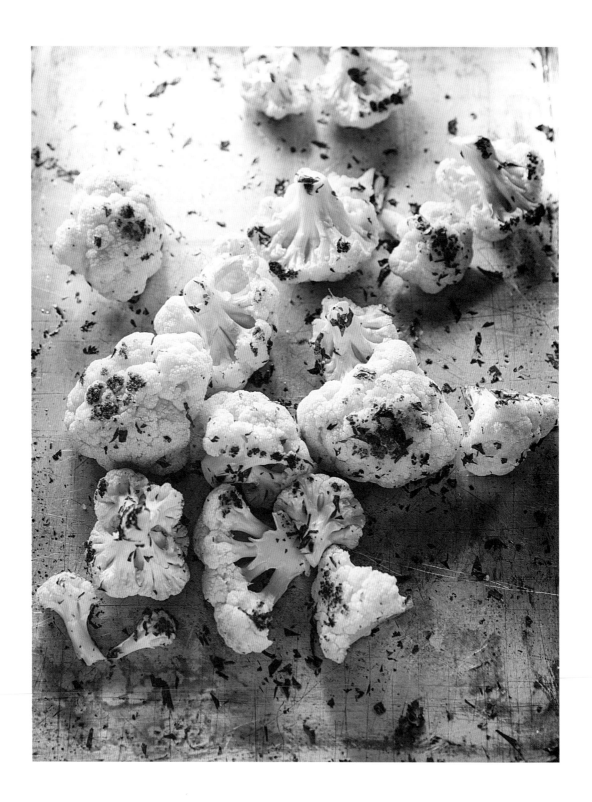

roasted cauliflower

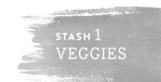

STASH 1
VEGGIES

2 heads cauliflower
1¼ tablespoons olive oil
2 tablespoons chopped cilantro
1 teaspoon Real Salt
1 teaspoon fresh-ground black pepper

1. Preheat oven to 350°F. Cut cauliflower into 1- to 2-inch chunks.

2. Place cauliflower on a baking sheet. Drizzle with olive oil, cilantro, salt, and pepper. Toss with your hands to coat well.

3. Roast for 15 minutes. Stir with a spatula, then roast for an additional 10 minutes or until a knife can easily pierce them.

4. Allow to cool, then transfer to a glass container.

gluten-free almond bread

2 cups blanched almond flour

2 tablespoons coconut flour (if you can't find this, use ¼ cup additional almond flour instead)

¼ cup ground flaxseed

½ teaspoon baking soda

½ teaspoon sea salt

5 large eggs

1½ tablespoons raw organic honey

1 tablespoon olive oil

1 tablespoon apple cider vinegar

1. Preheat oven to 325°F. Grease a small loaf pan.

2. In a food processor, combine flours, flaxseed, baking soda, and sea salt. Add wet ingredients. Pulse about 5 times to blend.

3. Pour batter into the greased pan. It should fill it about halfway.

4. Bake for 20 minutes, then cover with foil and return to the oven for another 10 minutes, or until a toothpick inserted in the middle comes out clean.

5. Cool bread for about 20 minutes, then remove from pan.

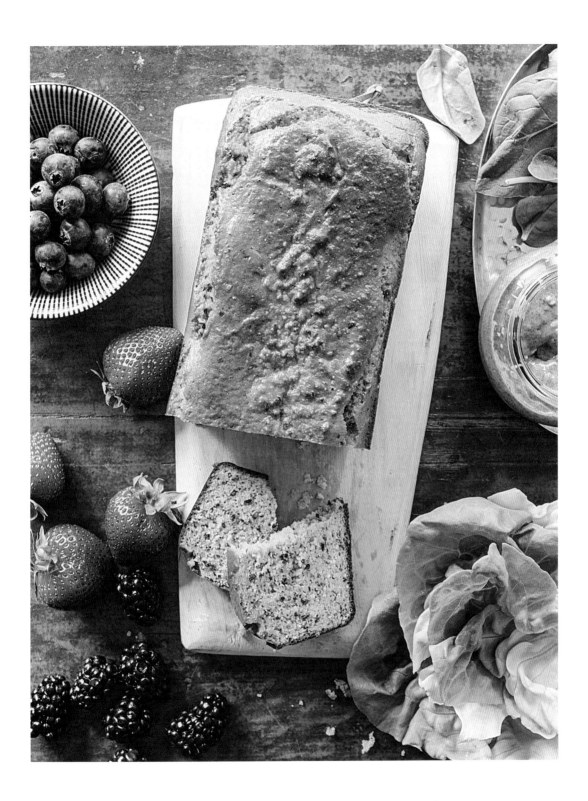

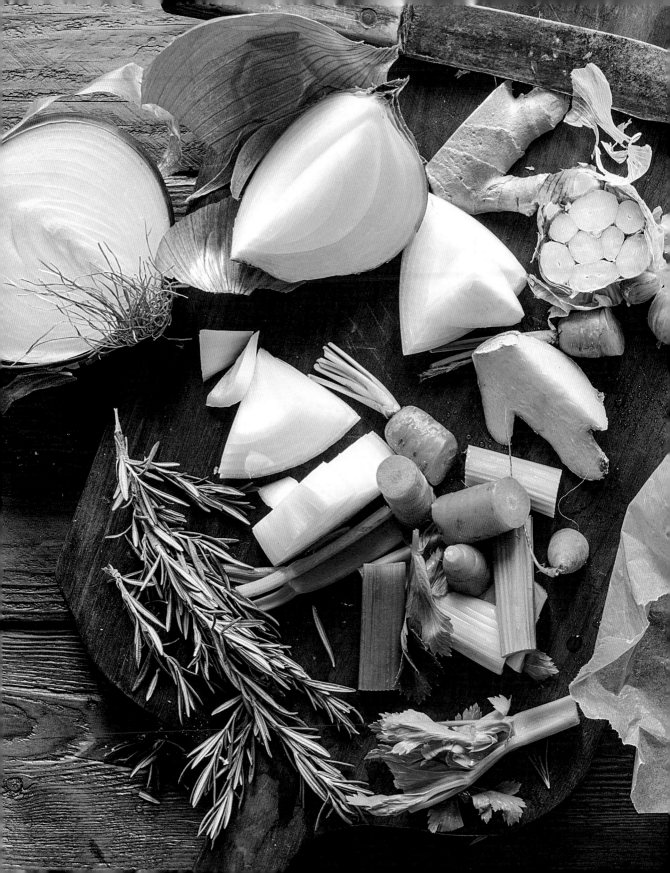

Broth Recipes

AND

Stashes

2 THROUGH 6

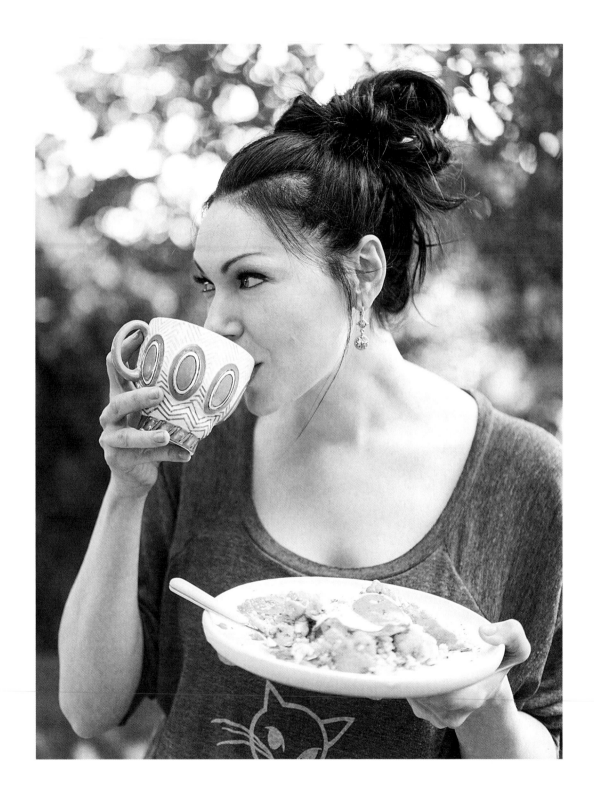

THIS IS ONE OF OUR
FAVORITE SECTIONS IN THE BOOK—

the recipes! Time to pull your slow cooker out of storage, because you're going to need it. In *Chapter 10,* you'll see how unbelievably easy it is to make beef, chicken, fish, and vegetable broth. *Chapter 11* has five stashes, each containing a broth, protein, carbs, veggies, and snacks, all mouth-watering recipes *low in calories* and high in flavor and nutrition. We'll teach you how to put it all together with our *three-week menu plan* full of new and exciting ways to build your meals!

BROTH
Recipes

chapter 10

Broths are potent tonics that are easily assimilated and absorbed by your body, and they are guaranteed to fill you up with maximum deliciousness and minimal calories. In this chapter, you'll find the recipes for beef, chicken, wing, fish, and vegetarian broths referenced earlier in the book. They're all loaded with micronutrients and truly are optimum nutrition in a bowl.

ANYONE CAN MAKE BROTH

LAURA: I was always afraid of making broths because it seemed as though you had be a classically trained French chef in a kitchen, stirring up some complicated concoction in a big scary pot over a hot stove for hours. However, I found that broth is actually one of the easiest foods to make! And with the Stash Plan we make it even easier; prep only takes about ten minutes, max, and the more rough-hewn the ingredients, the better!

Whenever you make broth, cooking the bones as long as possible is what you want to strive for. (The exception to this is the fish broth, which can be cooked for a shorter amount of time due to the tiny bones in the fish!) This long cooking time is what allows you to extract the maximum nutrients, collagen, marrow, and cartilage from the bones. Here are some of our favorite tips:

- Use a slow cooker. I'm obsessed with my slow cooker. When moving back to New York for season four of *Orange Is the New Black*, the first thing I pulled out of a moving box was my slow cooker so I could get a beef bone broth simmering right away. Slow cookers are ideal for broth, as they have controlled, steady heat and are designed to be safe to use even when you aren't home. Simply put all the ingredients in the slow cooker in the morning, turn it on high for eight to ten hours, and you'll come home to a wonderful aroma and a pot full of nourishing broth. You can also start the broth before you go to bed and leave it on all night. If I know I'm going to cook the broth for a whole night, I start it on low, then will move up to high the last few hours.

- When using a soup pot, once the broth starts to boil, turn to low and cook covered for eight hours. I usually use my soup pot when I know I'll be working at home.

- Because broths freeze so well, it's easy to make an enormous pot and then store it for later use to drink for your tonic or to cook with.

basic beef broth

1 pound organic grass-fed marrowbones

1 pound organic grass-fed knucklebones

1 pound bone-in short rib, (optional, but we suggest using it)

2 large carrots

2 stalks celery

1 head garlic

2-ounce chunk fresh ginger

2 sprigs fresh rosemary

2 sprigs fresh thyme

1 large yellow onion

2 teaspoons Real Salt (or sea salt of your choice)

2 teaspoons black peppercorns

1. Place bones in a large slow cooker.

2. Rinse off carrots, celery, garlic, ginger, and herbs. You don't have to dry them because they are going right into the slow cooker to be covered with water.

3. Chop ends off carrots and celery, then chop into large chunks. Chop ends off onion, peel off outside layer, then chop into big chunks. Slice the head of garlic in half. Slice ginger length-wise—no need to peel it. These don't have to look perfect. The less time you spend, the better! Add to cooker.

3. Sprinkle herbs, salt, and peppercorns on top. Cover with water to 2 inches above the bones and veggies. Set the slow cooker on high and cook for at least 15 hours. You want a slow simmer; adjust accordingly.

(recipe continues)

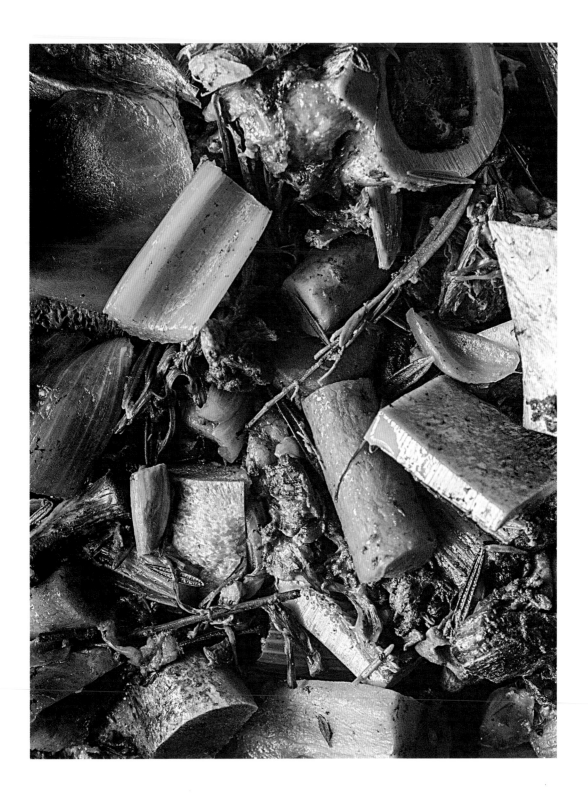

4. When broth is finished, allow it to cool slightly. Pour the broth through a strainer into another large bowl.

5. Transfer the strained broth to a glass container and put in the fridge. After the broth cools, it may be gelatinous; the amount of gelatin depends on the collagen content of the bones you used. This is a good thing! Whatever the gelatin content, this micronutrient-rich broth is still liquid vitamins for you, healing you from the inside out. Every time you make it, it will have its own unique texture, mouth feel, and taste.

6. Once the broth is cold, the fat will harden on the top, making it super-easy for you to scoop it off and discard. How lovely! What's left is the Fountain of Youth.

basic chicken broth

5-pound chicken
2 large carrots
2 large stalks celery
1 head garlic
2 sprigs fresh rosemary
2 sprigs fresh thyme
1 large yellow onion
2 teaspoons Real Salt (or sea salt of your choice)
2 teaspoons black peppercorns

1. Place chicken in a large slow cooker.

2. Rinse off carrots, celery, garlic, and herbs.

3. Chop ends off carrots and celery, then chop into large chunks. Chop ends off onion, peel off outside layer, then chop into big chunks. Slice the head of garlic in half. These don't have to look perfect. The less time you spend, the better! Add to cooker.

4. Sprinkle herbs, salt, and peppercorns on top. Cover with water to 2 inches above the chicken and veggies. Set the slow cooker on high and cook for about 12–15 hours. You want a slow simmer; adjust accordingly.

5. When broth is finished, allow it to cool slightly. Pour the broth through a strainer into another large bowl.

6. Transfer the strained broth to a glass container and put in the fridge.

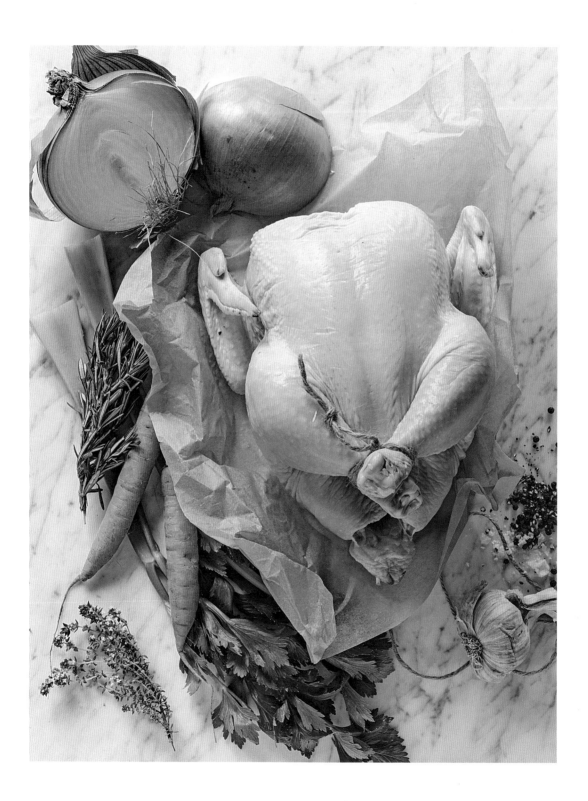

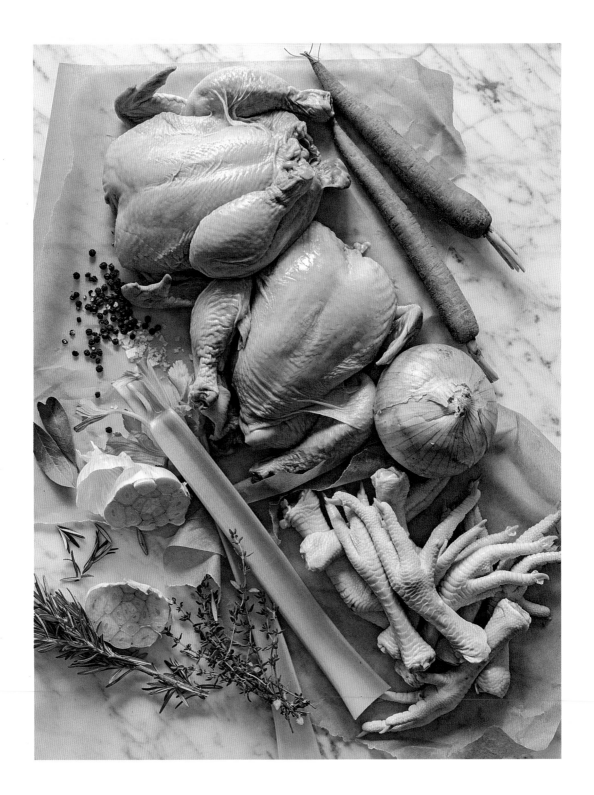

winged broth

2 2½ pound Cornish game hens
1 pound chicken feet
2 large carrots
2 stalks celery
1 head garlic
2 sprigs fresh rosemary
2 sprigs fresh thyme
1 large yellow onion
2 teaspoons Real Salt (or sea salt of your choice)
2 teaspoons black peppercorns

1. Place game hens and chicken feet in a large slow cooker.

2. Rinse off carrots, celery, garlic, and herbs.

3. Chop ends off carrots and celery, then chop into large chunks. Chop ends off onion, peel off outside layer, then chop into big chunks. Slice the head of garlic in half. These don't have to look perfect. The less time you spend, the better! Add to cooker.

4. Sprinkle herbs, salt, and peppercorns on top. Cover with water to 2 inches above the game hens, chicken feet, and veggies. Set the slow cooker on high and cook for 12–15 hours. You want a low simmer; adjust accordingly.

5. When broth is finished, allow it to cool slightly. Pour the broth through a strainer into another large bowl.

6. Transfer the strained broth to a glass container and put in the fridge.

basic fish broth

We like branzino for this broth, but any kind of whitefish works. Head, tail, scales, eyes, and all!! You'll note that this is our basic broth recipe with a few great additions: We add 1 parsnip to sweeten the broth, fresh basil to cut the fish taste, wakame for its nutrient-rich iodine and thyroid support, and bay leaves to make the broth more stock hearty. If you do add seaweed, be aware that it tends to be like those Magic Grow toys from when you were a kid, where you drop the small sponge animal into water and it grows to quickly become ten times its size! A little seaweed goes a very long way. Trust us, this broth is great!

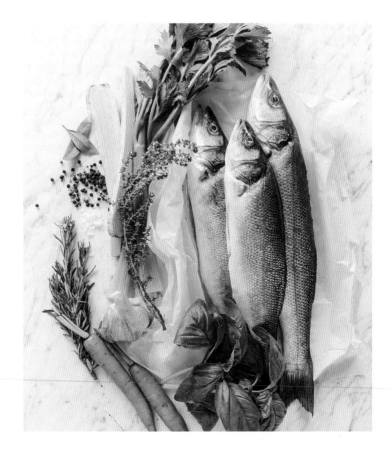

2 pounds whole branzino or several smaller fish

2 large carrots

2 large stalks celery

1 head garlic

2 sprigs fresh rosemary

2 sprigs fresh thyme

2 bay leaves

1 cup fresh basil

1 large yellow onion

1 large parsnip

¼ cup wakame

2 teaspoons Real Salt (or sea salt of your choice)

2 teaspoons black peppercorns

1. Place fish in large slow cooker.

2. Rinse off carrots, celery, garlic, herbs, and parsnip.

3. Chop ends off carrots, parsnip and celery, then chop into large chunks. Chop ends off onion, peel off outside layer, then chop into big chunks. Slice the head of garlic in half. These don't have to look perfect. The less time you spend, the better! Add to cooker.

4. Sprinkle herbs, seaweed, salt, and peppercorns on top. Cover with water to 2 inches above the fish and veggies. Set the slow cooker on high and cook for 6–12 hours. You want a low simmer; adjust accordingly.

5. When broth is finished, allow it to cool slightly. Pour the broth through a strainer into another large bowl.

6. Transfer the strained broth to a glass container and put in the fridge.

vegetable broth

This is an easy alternative to the meat and fish bone broths. There are no rules—you can literally add any kind of vegetables you enjoy. The more herbs, the better. We like to start with the basic veggies used in our bone broth recipes and go from there. Whatever you add will bump up the flavor and consistency, making the broth heartier in lieu of not using bones. Have fun experimenting!

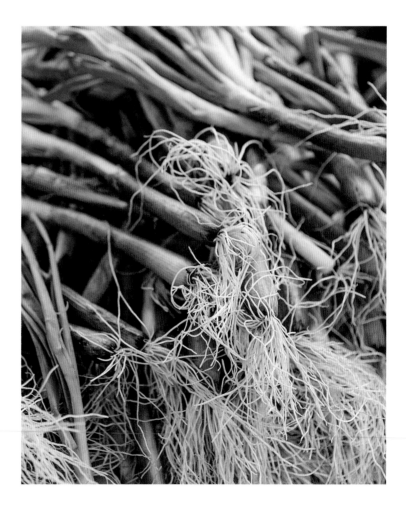

2 large carrots

2 large stalks celery

1 head garlic

VEGGIES OF YOUR CHOICE:

2 large tomatoes

¼ pound shiitake mushrooms

1–2 parsnips

1–2 turnips

1 bulb fennel

1–2 bay leaves

2 sprigs fresh rosemary

2 sprigs fresh thyme

1 large yellow onion

2 teaspoons Real Salt (or other sea salt of your choice)

2 teaspoons black peppercorns

1. Rinse off carrots, celery, garlic, any other veggies you are using, and herbs.

2. Chop ends off carrots and celery, then chop into large chunks. Chop ends off onion, peel off outside layer, then chop into big chunks. Chop any other veggies into chunks. Slice top off garlic— you don't have to peel or separate the cloves. These don't have to look perfect. The less time you spend, the better! Add to cooker.

3. Sprinkle herbs, salt, and peppercorns on top. Cover with water to 2 inches above the veggies. Set the slow cooker on low and cook for 6–12 hours. You want a low simmer; adjust accordingly.

4. When broth is finished, allow it to cool slightly. Pour the broth through a strainer into another large bowl.

5. Transfer the strained broth to a glass container and put in the fridge.

chapter 11

Stashes
2 THROUGH 6

Ready to keep on Stashing? Let's go!

Before You Start

- **Use organic ingredients** as much as possible and always use real food ingredients—butter, for example, not margarine.

- **We love to cook with olive oil.** Cold-pressed oil retains more of the nutritive value.

- **Always use real salt,** not salt substitutes, as many of them contain MSG and other chemicals. Like olive oil, different salts have unique tastes. Real Salt, a brand of sea salt, is intensely flavorful, so we prefer it. You might also like to try Himalayan Pink Salt, which Laura is partial to, as it provides essential minerals and helps to balance electrolytes and your body's pH. It also aids in relaxing your muscles along with your mind.

- **Grind your own fresh peppercorns**—it makes a big difference.

Substitutions

- We particularly like butter lettuce for its flavor and adaptability for salad or a wrap, but feel free to use any green leafy lettuce of your choice.

- Persian cucumbers are very tasty and crunchy, so we prefer them, but you can replace with regular cucumbers.

- For fish, you can use any firm white fish that's wild-caught. Some people are not crazy about the taste of certain fish, so you can, for example, swap salmon for a whitefish if you like.

- A vinegar you'll see often in the recipes is ume plum vinegar. We like it because it is highest in antioxidants, and helps to kill off foreign substances in the blood. You can always swap for apple cider vinegar, but try ume plum vinegar because it tastes great and is a secret flavor weapon!

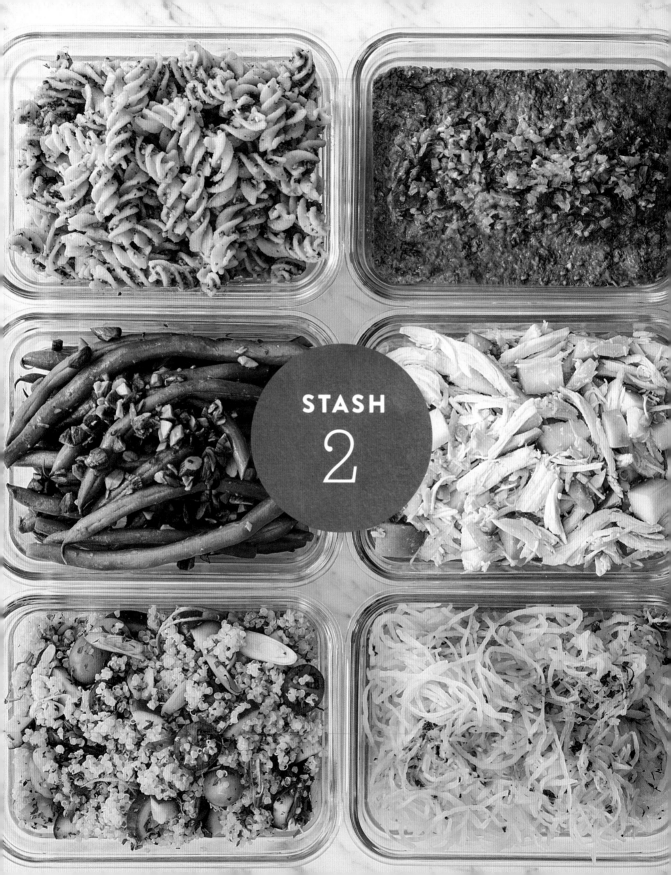

STASH

2

STASH 2

BROTH
- Basic Chicken Broth (page 198)

PROTEIN
- Chicken Salad
- Meat Loaf

CARBS
- Cilantro Pesto Brown Rice Noodles
- Quinoa Tabbouleh

VEGGIES
- Green Beans Almondine
- Roasted Spaghetti Squash

HAND GRABBERS
- almond butter
- almonds
- Hass avocado
- blueberries
- butter lettuce
- dried coconut flakes
- eggs
- Gluten-Free Almond Bread (page 186)
- Granny Smith apples
- spinach
- walnuts

STASH 2: SHOPPING LIST

- 1 bunch of cilantro
- 1 pound ground beef
- 1 pound ground lamb
- 5 pound whole chicken
- 3 Granny Smith apples
- 4 cups (1½ pounds) green beans
- 1 spaghetti squash
- 1 large yellow onion
- 1 lemon
- 2 medium tomatoes
- 1 Persian cucumber
- 16-ounce carton of grape tomatoes
- 1 bunch of scallions
- 12 eggs
- 1 Hass avocado
- 2 heads of garlic

LEFT OVER FOR NEXT STASH
- ½ lemon
- approximately 6 scallions
- 5 eggs
- ¼ cup grape tomatoes

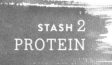

**STASH 2
PROTEIN**

chicken salad

Chicken meat from one 5-pound chicken (used from your broth)
1 large carrot
1 large celery stalk
1 tablespoon ume plum vinegar
1 tablespoon olive oil
2 teaspoons lemon juice or Dijon mustard
½ Granny Smith apple, chopped into small pieces
Real Salt
Fresh-ground black pepper

1. Once chicken broth has been cooking for 2–3 hours and the meat is cooked through—you can tell this by the meat easily coming off the bones—using tongs or two forks, pull as much chicken off the bones as you can. It will be hot, so be careful.

2. Let cool slightly, then use 2 forks to gently pull both chicken breasts off of the bone and place in a bowl. Then pull as much dark meat from the thighs, back, and drumsticks as you can. Put the chicken bones back into the broth for additional cooking.

3. Chop carrot and celery and place in a bowl with vinegar, olive oil, and lemon juice or Dijon mustard.

4. When the chicken is cooled slightly, chop it into small pieces. Mix all of the ingredients together. Add salt and pepper to taste.

meat loaf

¾ head garlic

1 stalk celery

1 large yellow onion

1 tablespoon chopped flat-leaf Italian parsley

1 tablespoon olive oil

2 medium tomatoes

¼ cup beef broth

½ pound grass-fed ground chuck

½ pound grass-fed ground lamb

½ cup bread crumbs, made from Gluten-Free Almond Bread

1 egg, beaten

1 teaspoon Real Salt

1 teaspoon fresh-ground black pepper

1. Preheat oven to 275°F. Chop garlic, celery, onion, and parsley.

2. In a sauté pan, heat the olive oil, then cook the vegetables over medium-low heat for 5 minutes.

3. Chop the tomatoes, then add to pan and cook for an additional 3 minutes, stirring occasionally.

4. Take the pan off the heat, add the beef broth, and allow to cool slightly.

5. In a large bowl, combine meats, ¾ of the onion mixture, bread crumbs, egg, and salt and pepper. Gently mix. You can use a fork to mix and aerate, or use your hands. Do not overmix.

6. Fill meat loaf pan with the mixture. Gently pat into the mold. Use your fingers to make a trough about 6 inches long and 2 inches wide, down the middle of the top. Fill it with the remaining onion mixture.

7. Cook for one hour, or until a meat thermometer reads 150–160 degrees and the meat loaf is cooked through.

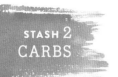

cilantro pesto brown rice noodles

1 teaspoon salt

3 cups brown rice noodles

PESTO

¼ cup plus 1 teaspoon olive oil

½ cup walnuts

½ cup pine nuts

1 cup cilantro

¼ cup parsley

1 garlic clove

¼ cup plus ½ tablespoon olive oil

⅓ teaspoon sea salt

½ teaspoon fresh-cracked black pepper

1 tablespoon fresh-squeezed lemon juice

1. Heat water to a boil with 1 teaspoon salt. Add noodles. Cook for 10 minutes. Noodles should be slightly al dente.

2. Transfer to a strainer and rinse with cold water to stop pasta from cooking. Shake off excess water and drizzle with a little olive oil to prevent sticking. Transfer to a glass container.

Pesto

1. Heat ½ tablespoon olive oil in a skillet. Add walnuts and pine nuts and toast until golden brown, stirring often. Let cool.

2. In a Vitamix blender, or another kind of powerful blender, add cilantro, parsley, garlic, ¼ cup olive oil, salt, pepper, and lemon juice. Add cooled nuts. Blend to a smooth consistency.

3. Pour over pasta and toss until mixed.

quinoa tabbouleh

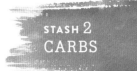

1 cup quinoa

2 tablespoons plain Greek yogurt

3 cups water, divided

½ cup broth (chicken or beef)

1 teaspoon Real Salt

2 tablespoon olive oil

1 tablespoon fresh-squeezed lemon juice

2 scallions

1 Persian cucumber, chopped

¼ cup chopped mint, lightly packed

¼ cup chopped parsley, lightly packed

1 cup grape tomatoes

Sea salt

Fresh-ground black pepper

• • • • •

LAURA

• • • • •

You can use a regular cucumber, but I like to scoop out the seeds when using a bigger cucumber for this recipe.

1. The night before serving, place quinoa in a glass bowl. Add yogurt and 1½ cups water. Mix until the yogurt is dissolved. Leave on the counter overnight. (This ferments the quinoa and predigests it, so you can digest it more easily.)

2. The next day, rinse the quinoa in a strainer until the water runs clear.

3. Place the quinoa in a 4-quart saucepan. Add broth, 1½ cups water, and salt. Cook on high until the quinoa begins to boil, then lower the flame, cover, and simmer for 15 minutes, stirring occasionally.

4. Place quinoa in a bowl with olive oil, lemon juice, scallions, chopped cucumber, mint, parsley, and grape tomatoes. Gently combine. Add salt and pepper to taste.

green beans almondine

4 cups green beans
Pinch of baking soda
1 tablespoon butter
⅓ cup chopped almonds
Sea salt
Fresh-ground black pepper

1. Heat 3 to 4 cups water to a boil.

2. Add green beans and a pinch of baking soda to bring out the vibrant green color. Blanch 2 minutes.

3. Strain beans and immediately rinse with cold water.

4. Melt butter in a pan, add almonds, and toast for 2 minutes, stirring constantly.

5. Turn off heat, add green beans, and toss. Add salt and pepper to taste.

roasted spaghetti squash

1 spaghetti squash
¼ bunch fresh cilantro
Sea salt
Fresh-ground black pepper
½ tablespoon olive oil

1. Preheat oven to 350°F. Cut spaghetti squash in half, scoop out seeds from both halves, and discard. Place squash cut side up on a baking sheet or in a roasting pan

2. Finely chop cilantro and sprinkle over the squash. Season with salt and pepper and drizzle olive oil over the edges and on the inside. Use your fingers or the back of a spoon to spread evenly.

3. Roast for 45 minutes, until the edges are browned and a fork goes through smoothly.

4. Let cool. If there is liquid inside the squash, do not remove. The squash will soak it back up and it helps to keep the flesh moist.

5. When cool, take a fork and pull the squash out from front to back. It will look like spaghetti.

STASH 2: MEAL PLAN

Thursday

MEAL 1
- ½ cup Quinoa Tabbouleh
- 1 cup Green Beans Almondine
- 2 fried eggs

Snack
- 1 Granny Smith apple
- 10 walnuts

MEAL 2
- 4 ounces Meat Loaf
- 1 cup Green Beans Almondine
- ½ cup Cilantro Pesto Brown Rice Noodles

Snack
- 1 cup blueberries
- 10 almonds
- 1 tablespoon coconut flakes

  Use 1 teaspoon of brown rice syrup to add sweetness.

MEAL 3
- 4 ounces Chicken Salad (place on top of leftover spinach from Stash 1, drizzle with olive oil and ume plum vinegar)
- 1 cup Roasted Spaghetti Squash
- ½ cup Quinoa Tabbouleh

Friday

MEAL 1
- 2 eggs scrambled in 1 tablespoon real butter
- 2 slices almond bread avocado toast

  Place eggs on top.

  Place a piece of butter lettuce over each piece.

Snack
- 1 Granny Smith apple, sliced and sprinkled with cinnamon, if desired
- 2 tablespoons almond butter

MEAL 2
- 4 ounces Meat Loaf
- 1 cup Green Beans Almondine
- ½ cup Cilantro Pesto Brown Rice Noodles

Snack
- 1 cup blueberries
- 2 tablespoons sunflower seeds
- 1 tablespoon coconut flakes

MEAL 3
- 4 ounces Chicken Salad
- 1 cup Roasted Spaghetti Squash
- ½ cup Quinoa Tabbouleh

Saturday

MEAL 1

- 2 scrambled eggs in 1 tablespoon real butter with 1 cup spinach
- ½ cup Quinoa Tabbouleh
- ½ Hass avocado

Snack

- 1 cup blueberries
- 2 tablespoons sunflower seeds
- 1 tablespoon coconut flakes

MEAL 2

- 4 ounces Chicken Salad
- 1 cup Green Beans Almondine
- ½ cup Cilantro Pesto Brown Rice Noodles

Snack

- 1 Granny Smith apple, sliced and sprinkled with cinnamon, if desired
- 2 tablespoons almond butter

MEAL 3

- 4 ounces Meat Loaf
- ½ cup Quinoa Tabbouleh
- 1 cup Roasted Spaghetti Squash

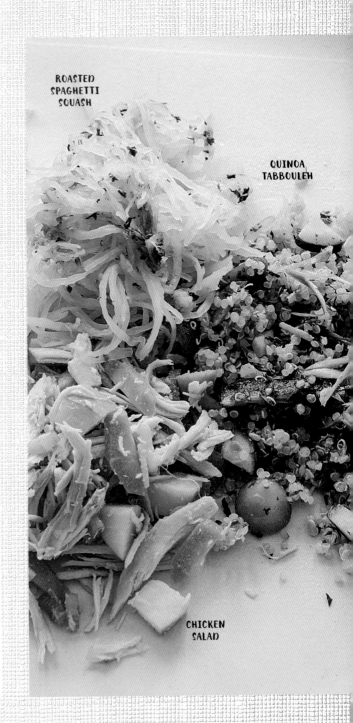

ROASTED
SPAGHETTI
SQUASH

QUINOA
TABBOULEH

CHICKEN
SALAD

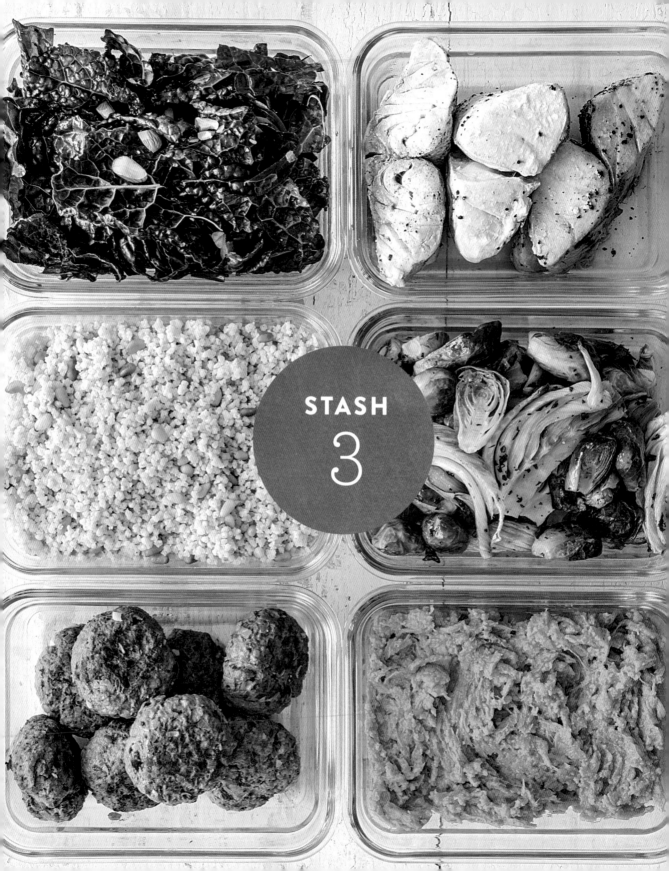

STASH

3

STASH 3

BROTH

- Fish (page 202)

PROTEIN

- Grass-fed Sliders
- Parcel-Poached Sea Bass

CARBS

- Nutty Millet
- Mashed Sweet Potatoes

VEGGIES

- Marinated Kale Salad
- Roasted Brussels Sprouts with Fennel

HAND GRABBERS

- almond butter
- almonds
- Hass avocado
- blueberries
- butter lettuce
- dried coconut flakes
- eggs
- Gluten-Free Almond Bread (page 186)
- Granny Smith apples
- spinach
- walnuts

STASH 3: SHOPPING LIST

- 1 pound ground beef
- 2 heads of garlic
- 1 bunch of cilantro
- 12 eggs
- 3 wild-caught sea bass fillets (approximately 6 ounces each)
- 5 shallots (or enough for ½ cup)
- 2 cups brussels sprouts
- 1 bunch of Italian flat leaf parsley
- 1 large head of fennel
- 2 large sweet potatoes
- 2 large bunches of kale
- 1 lemon
- 2 Hass avocados
- 6-ounce container of blueberries
- 3 Granny Smith apples

- 2 pounds whole branzino
- 2 large carrots
- 2 large stalks celery
- 2 sprigs fresh rosemary
- 2 sprigs fresh thyme
- 2 bay leaves
- 1 cup fresh basil
- 1 large yellow onion
- 1 large parsnip
- ¼ cup wakame

LEFT OVER FOR NEXT STASH

- 11 eggs
- ½ bunch flat-leaf Italian parsley
- ½ head of garlic
- Approximately ½ cup cilantro

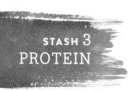

grass-fed sliders

½ cup chopped shallots
2 minced garlic cloves
1 tablespoon chopped parsley
1½ tablespoons olive oil
1 pound grass-fed ground beef
½ teaspoon salt
½ teaspoon fresh-ground black pepper
4 tablespoons broth

1. Chop the shallots, garlic, and parsley.

2. Heat 1 tablespoon olive oil in a pan over medium heat. Sauté shallots and garlic until the shallots are translucent, about 5 minutes. Allow to cool.

3. In a bowl, gently mix ground beef, shallot, garlic, parsley, salt, and pepper. Shape into 2-ounce patties/sliders.

4. Heat ½ tablespoon olive oil in a pan over medium heat. Cook 1 batch of sliders. Add 2 tablespoons broth. Cover and let cook for 2–3 minutes. Flip, then add 2 more tablespoons broth. Cover and cook for 3 minutes.

5. Repeat with second batch.

parcel-poached sea bass

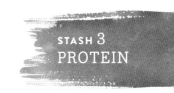
3 sea bass fillets, each weighing about 6 ounces

1½ tablespoons olive oil

1½ tablespoons fresh-squeezed lemon juice

Sea salt

Fresh-ground black pepper

1. Line 3 sheets of tinfoil with parchment paper and place fish in the middle.

2. Top each filet with ½ tablespoon olive oil, ½ tablespoon lemon juice, and salt and pepper to taste.

3. Wrap each fillet as in a pouch, rolling foil down and sides up.

4. Place in a dry, clean skillet and cook for 8–10 minutes on medium-low or until the fish is opaque.

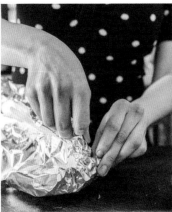
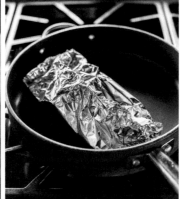
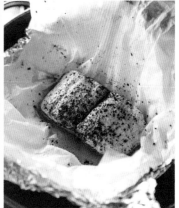

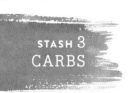

**STASH 3
CARBS**

nutty millet

4 tablespoons olive oil

1 cup millet

2 cups water

½ cup pine nuts

4 garlic cloves, finely chopped

1. In a sauté pan, heat 2 tablespoons olive oil over medium heat. Add millet. Sauté for 7–10 minutes, stirring frequently, until millet is slightly browned.

2. Pour millet into a saucepan and add water. Boil on medium-high for 25 minutes.

3. In the same sauté pan, heat 2 tablespoons olive oil over medium heat. Add pine nuts. Toast, stirring frequently, for 2–3 minutes. (They toast very quickly!)

4. When millet is tender, combine with pine nuts.

marinated kale salad

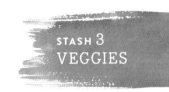

8 cups kale
Juice of ½ lemon
2 tablespoons olive oil
1 teaspoon Real Salt

1. Wash kale and dry. Cut the spine off by slicing down on either side of it. Rip kale into bite-size pieces and transfer to a glass container.

2. Pour lemon juice, olive oil, and salt over the greens, and massage in well. Cover and put in the fridge.

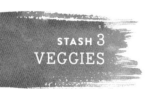

STASH 3
VEGGIES

roasted brussels sprouts with fennel

1 pound brussels sprouts
1 head fennel
¼ cup fresh cilantro
Sea salt
Fresh-ground black pepper
1 tablespoon olive oil

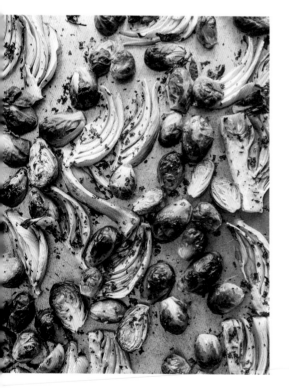

1. Preheat oven to 350°F. Trim tails of the sprouts and then cut in half. Cut fronds off fennel and discard, then thinly slice the bulb. Finely chop the cilantro.

2. Place sprouts and fennel on a baking sheet or roasting pan, then sprinkle cilantro, salt, and pepper on top. Drizzle on olive oil and mix all ingredients well with your hands.

3. Roast for 20 minutes, stir well, then roast for another 15 minutes. Allow to cool, then transfer to a glass container.

mashed sweet potatoes

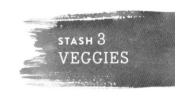

2 large sweet potatoes
1 tablespoon olive oil
Sea salt
Fresh-ground black pepper

1. Preheat oven to 350°F. Rub the outside of the sweet potatoes with olive oil.

2. Place on a baking sheet and cook for 50 minutes, or until a fork easily goes through.

3. Allow to cool. Pull skin off sweet potato; it should easily come off. Mash sweet potatoes with a fork and add salt and pepper to taste.

STASH 3: MEAL PLAN

Monday

MEAL 1

- Nutty Millet
- 1 cup blueberries
- 1 tablespoon coconut flakes

  Drizzle with 1 teaspoon real maple syrup.

Snack

- 1 Granny Smith apple
- 2 tablespoons almond butter

MEAL 2

- 3 Grass-fed Sliders
- 1 cup Roasted Brussels Sprouts with Fennel
- ½ cup Mashed Sweet Potatoes

Snack

- 1 slice toasted Gluten-Free Almond Bread
- 1 tablespoon real butter
- 1 teaspoon raw honey
- ½ cup blueberries

MEAL 3

- 4 ounces Parcel-Poached Sea Bass
- 2 cups Marinated Kale Salad
- ½ cup Nutty Millet

  Top with ½ avocado

Tuesday

MEAL 1

- 3 Grass-fed Sliders
- 1 fried egg
- ½ Hass avocado
- ¼ remaining grape tomatoes

  Cut in half and top the sliders.

Snack

- 1 slice toasted Gluten-Free Almond Bread
- 1 tablespoon almond butter

MEAL 2

- 4 ounces Parcel-Poached Sea Bass
- 1 cup Roasted Brussels Sprouts with Fennel
- ½ cup Mashed Sweet Potatoes

Snack

- 1 Granny Smith apple
- 1 tablespoon sunflower seeds

MEAL 3

- 3 Grass-fed Sliders
- ½ cup Nutty Millet
- 2 cups Marinated Kale Salad
- ½ Hass avocado
- 2 cups butter lettuce

  Wrap sliders in butter lettuce and top with avocado.

Wednesday

MEAL 1

- ½ cup Nutty Millet
- 1 chopped Granny Smith apple
- 1 teaspoon real maple syrup

Snack

- 1 cup blueberries
- 2 tablespoons sunflower seeds
- 1 tablespoon coconut flakes

MEAL 2

- 3 Grass-fed Sliders
- 2 cups Marinated Kale Salad with 10 chopped almonds
- ½ Hass avocado

Snack

- 1 slice toasted Gluten-Free Almond Bread
- 1 tablespoon real butter
- 1 teaspoon raw honey

MEAL 3

- 4 ounces Parcel-Poached Sea Bass
- 1 cup Roasted Brussels Sprouts with Fennel
- ½ cup Mashed Sweet Potatoes
- 2 cups butter lettuce

  Wrap sea bass in butter lettuce and top with sweet potatoes.

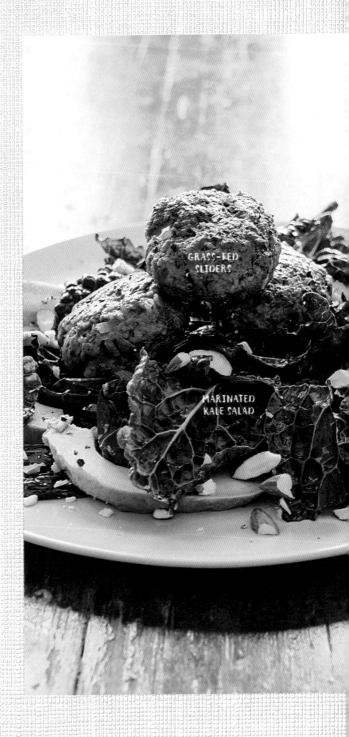

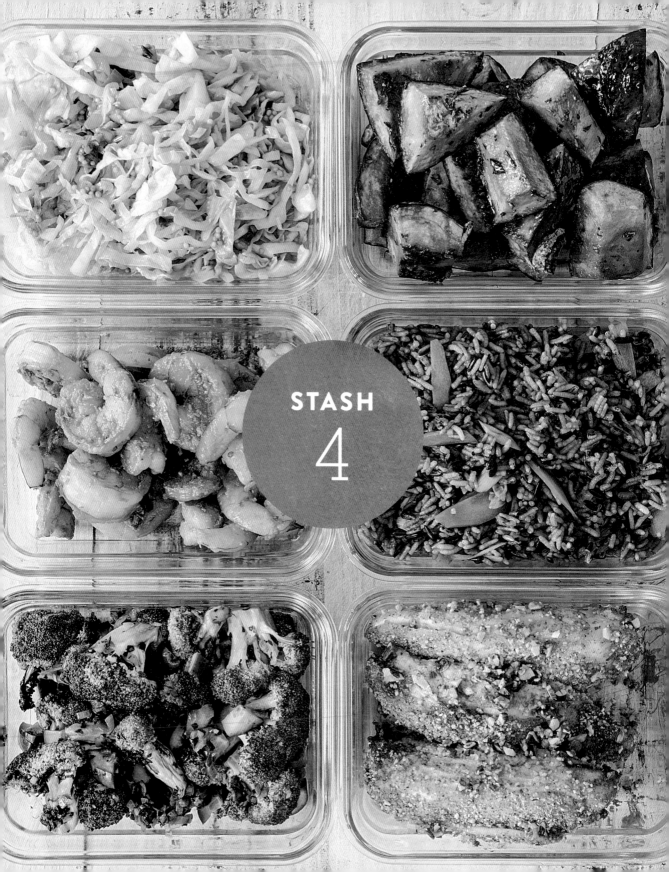

STASH

4

STASH 4

BROTH

- Winged Broth (page 201)

PROTEIN

- Coconut Almond Chicken
- Ginger Shrimp

CARBS

- Purple Rice Stir-Fry
- Kabocha Squash

VEGGIES

- Broccoli Salad
- Curried Cabbage

HAND GRABBERS

- almond butter
- almonds
- Hass avocado
- blackberries
- butter lettuce
- dried coconut flakes
- eggs
- Gluten-Free Almond Bread (page 186)
- Granny Smith apples
- spinach
- walnuts

STASH 4: SHOPPING LIST

- 1 large shallot
- 3 bone-in chicken breasts
- 1 pound shelled, deveined shrimp
- 2 Hass avocados
- 2 containers of blackberries
- 1½-pound bag of carrots (approximately 10–12)
- 1 head of broccoli
- 1 Persian cucumber
- 1 small cabbage
- 2 large yellow onions
- 1 kabocha squash
- 1 small white onion
- 1 lemon
- 2 Granny Smith apples
- 1 bunch of thyme
- 1 bunch of rosemary
- 2 2½ pound Cornish game hens
- 1 pound chicken feet
- 2 stalks celery
- 1 head garlic

LEFT OVER FOR NEXT STASH

- ½ Hass avocado
- 3 carrots
- ½ lemon
- ¾ bunch of rosemary
- ⅗ bunch of thyme

coconut almond chicken

COCONUT MILK

4 cups water

2 cups unsweetened shredded coconut

CHICKEN

3 bone-in 5-ounce chicken breasts

2 cups almond flour

2 teaspoons Real Salt

1 teaspoon pepper

1 teaspoon cumin

1 teaspoon paprika

1 teaspoon cayenne pepper

1 teaspoon garlic powder

1 cup chopped almonds

1. Make the coconut milk: Heat water to a simmer, not a full boil. Pour hot water and coconut into a blender and blend until smooth.

2. Pour mixture through a nut bag or cheesecloth. Make sure you have a bowl underneath to catch the milk. Squeeze the nut bag or cheesecloth with your hands to get liquid to strain through. Once all of the liquid is squeezed out, discard remaining mixture. Place 2 cups of your homemade coconut milk into a bowl and add the chicken breasts.

3. Marinate in the fridge for 30 minutes to an hour. (Save the remaining coconut milk for other recipes in this Stash.)

4. Preheat oven to 350°F. After chicken is finished marinating, mix almond flour and all of the seasonings in a bowl. Dredge chicken in the flour mixture, then place on a baking sheet. Press almonds on top of the chicken breasts evenly.

5. Bake chicken for 45 minutes, or until the juices run clear.

ginger shrimp

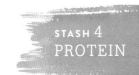

1 pound peeled, deveined raw shrimp

1½ tablespoons minced ginger

2 large garlic cloves

1 tablespoon Bragg Liquid Aminos (or high quality soy sauce)

2 tablespoons broth (chicken or beef)

1. Place all ingredients in a large sauté pan over medium heat. Cook shrimp for 5 minutes, or until the undersides are pink.

2. Flip over and cook for another 4 minutes or until shrimp is pink and fully cooked through.

purple rice stir-fry

2 cups purple rice (or brown rice), presoaked

3 tablespoons of plain Greek yogurt

3½ cups water

½ cup broth (chicken or beef)

½ cup plus 3 tablespoons homemade coconut milk (from Coconut Almond Chicken recipe)

⅓ cup chopped carrots

2 tablespoons scallions (left from Stash 2)

1 tablespoon Bragg Liquid Aminos (or high-quality soy sauce)

1 tablespoon ume plum vinegar

½ teaspoon Real Salt

1. The night before serving, place purple rice in a glass bowl. Add yogurt and 1½ cups of water. Mix until the yogurt is dissolved. Leave on the counter overnight. (This ferments the rice so it's easier to digest.)

2. The next day, rinse rice in a strainer until the water runs clear.

3. Bring 2 cups water, ½ cup broth, and ½ cup coconut milk to a boil in a saucepan.

4. Add rice and cook for 6–7 minutes or until the liquid is absorbed, but the rice is not mushy. We prefer a little al dente.

5. Allow to cool, then mix in carrots, scallions, Bragg Liquid Aminos, vinegar, 3 tablespoons coconut milk, and salt.

broccoli salad

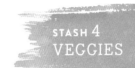

1 head broccoli
1 tablespoon olive oil
1 tablespoon shallots
1 tablespoon cilantro
1 teaspoon Real Salt
1 teaspoon fresh-ground black pepper
1 Persian or regular cucumber
1 teaspoon ume plum vinegar

1. Heat oven to 350°F. Chop broccoli head into pieces and place on a baking sheet. Chop shallots and cilantro.

2. Toss the broccoli with olive oil, shallots, cilantro, salt, and pepper. Roast for 10 minutes, then allow to cool.

3. Chop cucumber into small pieces. Toss roasted broccoli with vinegar and cucumbers.

STASH 4
VEGGIES

curried cabbage

1 small cabbage
1 small white onion
1 tablespoon olive oil
2 teaspoons mustard seed
1 teaspoon ground turmeric
Sea salt to taste
1 teaspoon fresh-squeezed lemon juice (optional)

1. Thinly slice cabbage. Dice onion.

2. In large skillet, heat oil, then add mustard seed and turmeric and allow to sizzle for a moment.

3. Add onion and sauté for several minutes, stirring frequently.

4. Add cabbage and mix thoroughly. Cook uncovered over medium heat, stirring continuously, until cabbage begins to wilt.

5. Salt to taste, and stir in lemon juice, if desired.

kabocha squash

1 kabocha squash
¼ cup flat-leaf Italian parsley
Sea salt
Fresh-ground black pepper
1½ tablespoons olive oil

1. Preheat oven to 350°F. Wash the squash really well, then cut into medium-sized chunks. Remove all seeds. Finely chop parsley.

2. Place squash on a baking sheet or roasting pan, then sprinkle parsley, salt, and pepper on top. Drizzle on olive oil and mix all ingredients well with your hands.

3. Roast for 15 minutes, stir squash, then roast for another 15 minutes.

4. Allow to cool, then transfer to a glass container.

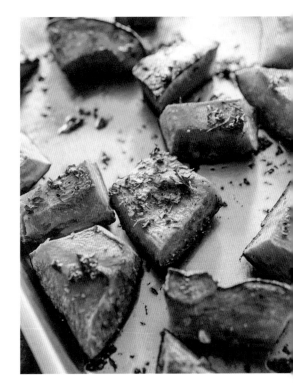

STASH 4: MEAL PLAN

Thursday

MEAL 1

- 2 slices Gluten-Free Almond Bread
- 1 teaspoon butter
- 2 scrambled eggs

Snack

- 1 Granny Smith apple
- 2 tablespoons almond butter

MEAL 2

- 4 ounces Coconut Almond Chicken
- ¼ cup Purple Rice Stir-fry
- 1 cup Curried Cabbage

Snack

- 1 cup blackberries
- ½ Hass avocado

MEAL 3

- 4 ounces Ginger Shrimp
- ½ cup Kabocha Squash
- 1 cup Broccoli Salad

Friday

MEAL 1

- ½ cup Purple Rice Stir-fry
- 1 egg
- ½ Hass avocado

Snack

- 1 cup blackberries
- 10 almonds
- 1 teaspoon coconut flakes

MEAL 2

- 4 ounces Ginger Shrimp
- 1 cup Broccoli Salad
- 2 cups butter lettuce
- ½ cup Kabocha Squash
- 10 chopped almonds
- 1 tablespoon olive oil

  Make a salad topped with shrimp, salad, and squash.

Snack

- ½ cup Kabocha Squash
- 1 Granny Smith apple, sliced and sprinkled with cinnamon, if desired

MEAL 3

- 4 ounces Coconut Almond Chicken
- ¼ cup Purple Rice Stir-fry
- 1 cup Curried Cabbage

Saturday

MEAL 1

- 1¼ cups broth
- 2 eggs
- 2 slices toasted Gluten-Free Almond Bread
- 1 teaspoon real butter

   Heat broth, drop the eggs into it. Stir, heating until eggs are cooked.

Snack

- 1 sliced Granny Smith apple
- ½ Hass avocado mashed on top with salt

MEAL 2

- 4 ounces Coconut Almond Chicken
- ½ cup Purple Rice Stir-fry
- 1 cup Broccoli Salad
- 2 cups butter lettuce
- 1 tablespoon sunflower seeds
- 1 tablespoon olive oil

   Chop chicken, then top lettuce with all the components.

Snack

- 1 slice toasted Gluten-Free Almond Bread
- 1 tablespoon almond butter
- 1 cup blackberries

MEAL 3

- 4 ounces Ginger Shrimp
- ½ cup Kabocha Squash
- 1 cup Curried Cabbage

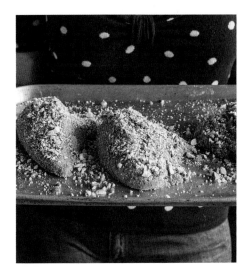

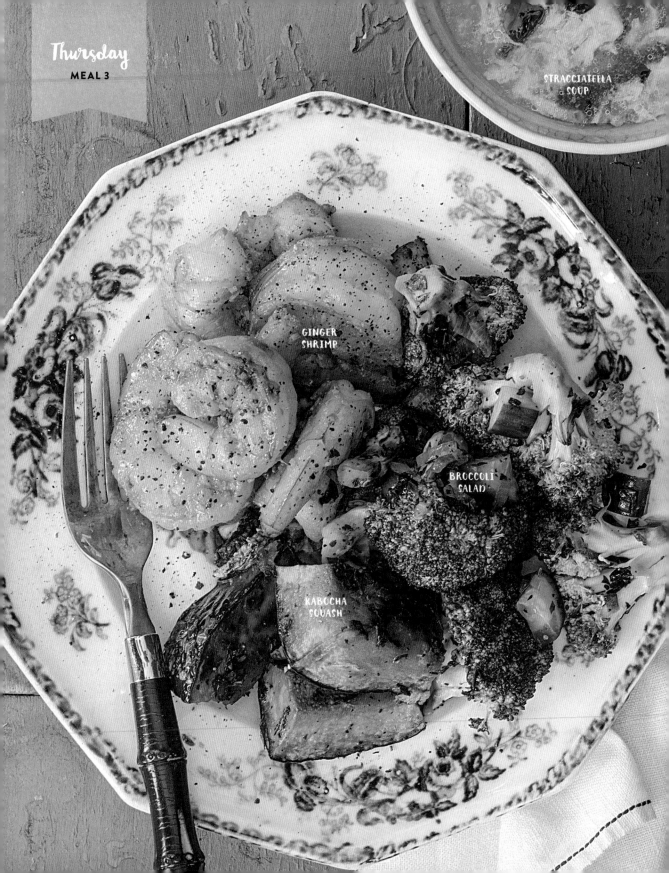

STRACCIATELLA
SOUP

GINGER
SHRIMP

BROCCOLI
SALAD

KABOCHA
SQUASH

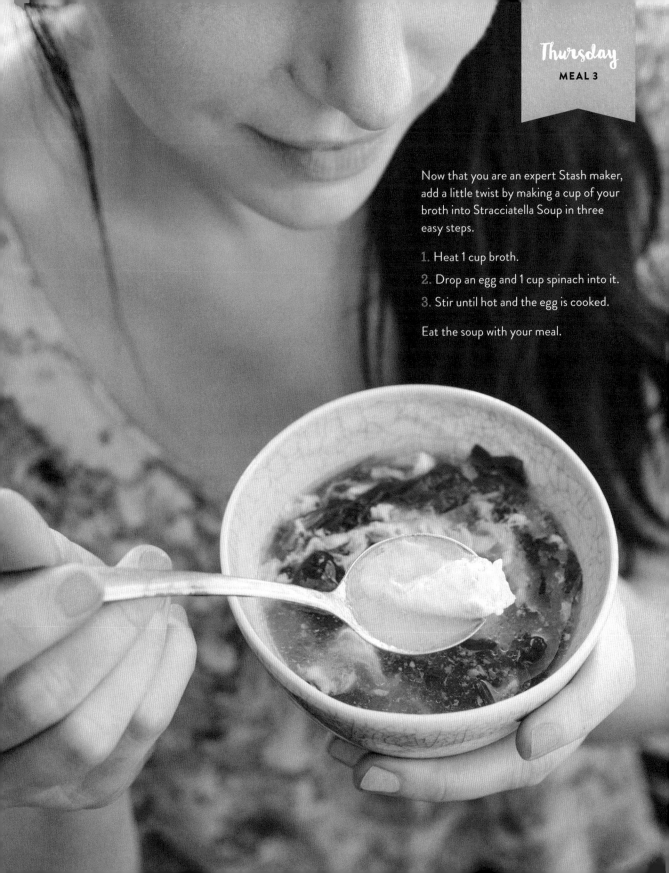

Now that you are an expert Stash maker, add a little twist by making a cup of your broth into Stracciatella Soup in three easy steps.

1. Heat 1 cup broth.
2. Drop an egg and 1 cup spinach into it.
3. Stir until hot and the egg is cooked.

Eat the soup with your meal.

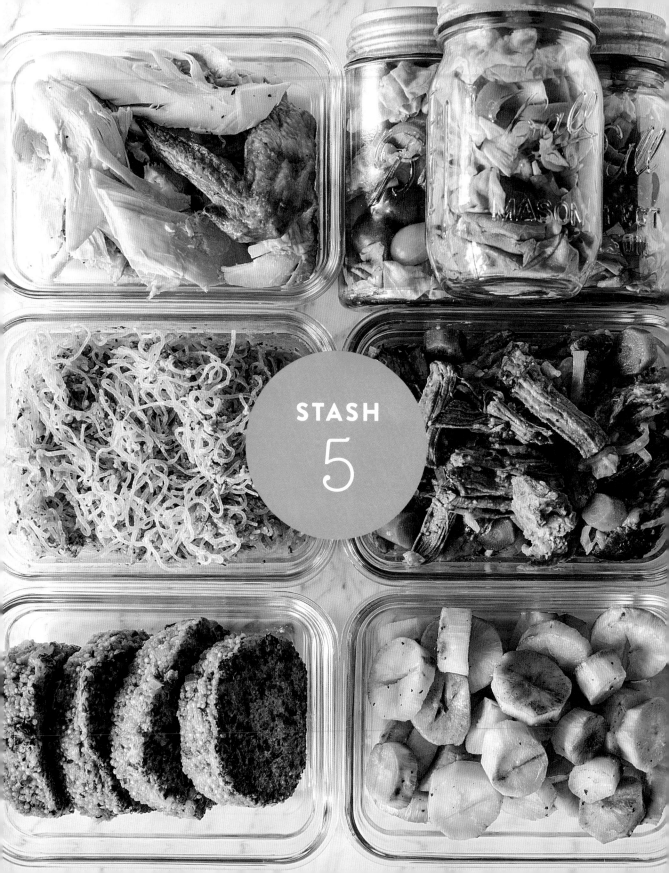

STASH

5

STASH 5

BROTH

- Winged Broth (page 201)

PROTEIN

- Pot Roast
- Roasted Chicken

CARBS

- Kelp Noodles with Cilantro Pesto
- Quinoa Patties

VEGGIES

- Salad Shakers
- Yucca Pucks

HAND GRABBERS

- almond butter
- almonds
- Hass avocado
- butter lettuce
- dried coconut flakes
- eggs
- Gluten-Free Almond Bread (page 186)
- Granny Smith apples
- spinach
- strawberries
- walnuts

STASH 5: SHOPPING LIST

- 1 pound beef roast
- 4 pounds chicken
- 3 heads of garlic
- 1 bunch of celery (approximately 8 stalks)
- 1 small orange
- 1 small bunch of cilantro
- 1 lemon
- 2 Persian cucumbers (or 1 large hothouse cucumber)
- 1 small white onion
- 2 large sweet potatoes
- 2 large yucca
- 2 large yellow onions
- 2 2½-pound Cornish game hens
- 1 pound chicken feet
- 3 butter lettuces
- 1 pound container of strawberries
- 12 eggs
- 1 bag of spinach
- 2 Hass avocados
- 2 Granny Smith apples

LEFT OVER FOR NEXT STASH

- 7 eggs
- 4 to 6 stalks of celery
- ½ lemon

pot roast

1 large yellow onion
6 garlic cloves, peeled
3 large carrots
1 pound beef roast
1 tablespoon sea salt
Fresh-ground black pepper
4 tablespoons olive oil
1 cup beef or chicken broth

1. Cut onion in half, then slice into half-moon pieces. Mince 4 garlic cloves, and slice the other 2 cloves into 4 pieces. Chop carrots into ½-inch chunks.

2. Slash 4 ½-inch-deep slices into the top of the roast, and insert the 4 garlic pieces. Sprinkle salt and pepper over the entire roast and rub in well.

3. Heat olive oil in a large Dutch oven, then sauté onion and minced garlic for 3 minutes. Push the mixture to sides of the pan and add roast. Brown on all sides.

4. Add carrots, broth, and enough water to cover the roast. Mix well with a spoon.

5. Cook, covered, for 2½–3 hours, or until the meat is tender and shreds easily with a fork.

roasted chicken

1 4-pound chicken
1 small orange
2 garlic cloves
2 sprigs rosemary
2 sprigs thyme
1 tablespoon olive oil
Sea salt
Fresh-cracked black pepper

1. Preheat oven 350°F. Cut orange into 2–3 slices and stuff into the cavity of the chicken, followed by the garlic cloves and herbs.

2. Pat chicken dry, then rub olive oil all over the outside. Sprinkle liberally with salt and pepper. Tie legs together with cooking twine. Tie wings close to the body. Place on a small rack on a baking sheet.

3. Cook for 1 hour, or until juices run clear. If the skin starts to get too golden brown before the hour is up, cover with tinfoil lined with natural parchment paper to prevent burning.

4. Allow chicken to cool until it's still warm to the touch, then pull meat away from the bones. (It's okay to play with your food, so use your hands!) Transfer to a glass container.

kelp noodles with cilantro pesto

1 12-ounce bag kelp noodles

PESTO
¼ cup plus ½ tablespoon olive oil
½ cup walnuts
½ cup pine nuts
1 cup cilantro
¼ cup parsley
1 garlic clove
⅓ teaspoon sea salt
½ teaspoon fresh-cracked pepper
1 tablespoon fresh-squeezed lemon juice

1. Drain the kelp noodles on paper towel and allow to dry. Place in a glass storage container.

Pesto

2. Heat ½ tablespoon olive oil in a skillet. Add walnuts and pine nuts and toast until golden brown, stirring often. Let cool.

3. In a Vitamix, or another powerful blender, add cilantro, parsley, garlic, ¼ cup olive oil, salt, pepper, and lemon juice. Add cooled nuts. Blend to a smooth consistency.

4. Pour over noodles and toss until mixed.

quinoa patties

1 cup quinoa

2 tablespoons plain yogurt

1 small onion

2 carrots

3 garlic cloves

2 large eggs

Sea salt and fresh-cracked pepper, to taste

2 tablespoons olive oil, plus more if needed

1 tablespoon chopped parsley

½ cup Mashed Sweet Potatoes

½ cup Gluten-Free Almond Bread bread crumbs

1. Soak quinoa for at least 2 hours in 2 tablespoons of plain yogurt. (You can also soak it overnight.)

2. Rinse quinoa in a strainer until the water runs clear. Place quinoa in a pot with 2 cups of water. Bring to a boil, then turn to low. Cook for about 15 minutes or until tender.

3. Dice onion and carrots. Mince garlic cloves.

4. Combine cooked quinoa, eggs, salt, and pepper in a large bowl.

5. Heat 1 tablespoon olive oil in a pan, then sauté onion, garlic, and carrots until onions are translucent.

6. Add parsley, sweet potatoes, and bread crumbs to quinoa mixture. Stir in onion, garlic, and carrots. Mix well until the texture is consistent.

7. Shape into 4 thick patties. Heat 1 tablespoon olive oil, then add patties. Cover, and cook over medium heat for 5 minutes. Flip patties over. Cover, and cook for 5 more minutes until patties are browned on each side and light in the middle.

salad shakers

2 heads of butter lettuce

2 carrots

2 celery stalks

2 Persian or regular cucumbers

DRESSING

4 tablespoons olive oil

Juice of ½ lemon

Sea salt

Fresh-ground black pepper

1. Rip lettuce into bite-size pieces. Chop carrots, celery, and cucumbers into small pieces.

2. Fill 3 medium mason jars with ingredients.

Dressing

3. Combine olive oil, lemon juice, and salt and pepper to taste.

4. Pour ⅓ of mixture into each mason jar.

yucca pucks

2 teaspoons Real Salt

2 large yucca

2 tablespoons olive oil

1 teaspoon fresh-cracked black pepper

1. Fill a pot with about 3 inches of water and 1 teaspoon salt and bring to a boil.

2. Peel yucca and cut into ¾-inch discs. Place in boiling water and cook for 7 minutes.

3. Preheat oven to 350°F. Drain yucca pucks and place on a baking sheet. Drizzle with the olive oil and rub in well with your hands. Rub oil into them well. Sprinkle with 1 teaspoon salt and pepper.

4. Roast for 7 minutes, flip each puck over with a spatula, then cook for another 7 minutes or until light golden brown.

5. Allow to cool, then transfer to a glass container.

Monday

MEAL 1

- 1 slice Gluten-Free Almond Bread
- 1 teaspoon butter
- 2 eggs, scrambled
- spinach salad with 1 tablespoon olive oil

Snack

- 1 cup strawberries
- 2 tablespoons raw sunflower seeds
- 1 teaspoon coconut flakes

MEAL 2

- 1 Quinoa Patty
- ½ Hass avocado
- 4 ounces Roasted Chicken
- Kelp Noodles with Cilantro Pesto

Snack

- 1 sliced Granny Smith apple
- 10 almonds

MEAL 3

- 1 cup Pot Roast
- 1 Salad Shaker
- 1 tablespoon olive oil
- 1 cup Yucca Pucks

Tuesday

MEAL 1

- 2 eggs
- 1 tablespoon real butter
- 2 cups spinach

  Cook spinach with eggs, making a scramble.

- 1 slice of toasted Gluten-Free Almond Bread

Snack

- 1 cup Yucca Pucks
- ½ Hass avocado

MEAL 2

- 1 cup Pot Roast
- 1 Salad Shaker
- Quinoa Patty

Snack

- 1 cup strawberries
- 2 tablespoons raw seeds
- 1 teaspoon coconut flakes

MEAL 3

- 4 ounces Roasted Chicken
- 1½ cups Kelp Noodles with Cilantro Pesto
- ½ Hass avocado
- 1 cup Yucca Pucks

Wednesday

MEAL 1

- 2 eggs
- 2 slices toasted Gluten-Free Almond Bread
- 1 teaspoon real butter
- ½ Hass avocado

Snack

- 1 Granny Smith apple
- 2 tablespoons almond butter

MEAL 2

- 1 Quinoa Patty
- 1½ cups Kelp Noodles with Cilantro Pesto
- 2 cups butter lettuce
- ½ Hass avocado

  Wrap chicken in lettuce and top with avocado.

Snack

- 1 cup strawberries
- 10 walnuts
- 1 teaspoon coconut flakes

MEAL 3

- 1 cup Pot Roast
- Salad Shaker
- 1 cup Yucca Pucks

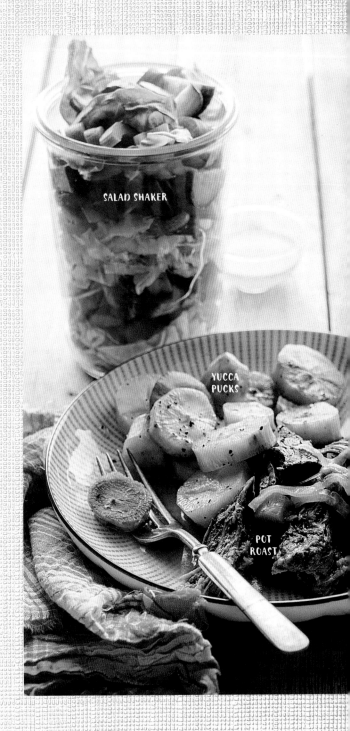

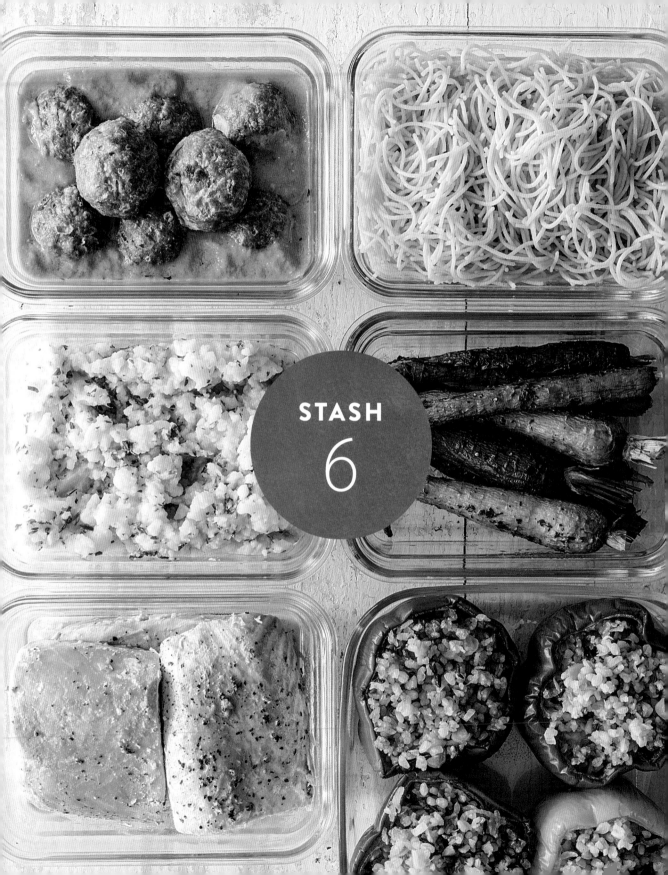

STASH
6

STASH 6

BROTH
- Basic Beef Broth (page 195)

PROTEIN
- Parcel-Poached Salmon
- Turkey Meatballs in Tomato Sauce

CARBS
- Quinoa Noodles
- Stuffed Peppers

VEGGIES
- Mashed Cauliflower
- Rainbow Carrots

HAND GRABBERS
- almond butter
- almonds
- Hass avocado
- blueberries
- butter lettuce
- dried coconut flakes
- eggs
- Gluten-Free Almond Bread (page 186)
- Granny Smith apples
- spinach
- walnuts

STASH 6: SHOPPING LIST

- 1 small white onion
- 3 fillets wild-caught salmon (approximately 6 ounces)
- 1 pound ground turkey
- 1 lemon
- 4 bell peppers (different colors)
- 2 large yellow onions
- 4 medium heirloom tomatoes
- 1 handful fresh basil
- 1 small bunch of fresh oregano
- 2 medium heads cauliflower
- 10 rainbow carrots
- 4 heads of garlic
- 2 cups spinach
- 1 head of butter lettuce
- 2 Hass avocados
- 2 Granny Smith apples
- 1 large container of blueberries
- 1 pound organic grass-fed marrowbones
- 1 pound organic grass-fed knucklebones
- 1 pound bone-in short ribs
- 2 large carrots
- 2 stalks celery
- 2-ounce chunk fresh ginger
- 2 sprigs fresh rosemary
- 2 sprigs fresh thyme
- 1 large yellow onion

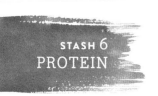

parcel-poached salmon

3 4-ounce fillets wild-caught salmon
1½ tablespoons olive oil
1½ tablespoons fresh-squeezed lemon juice
Sea salt to taste
Fresh-ground black pepper, to taste

1. Line 3 sheets of tinfoil with parchment paper and place fish in the middle.

2. Top each fillet with ½ tablespoon olive oil, ½ tablespoon lemon juice, and salt and pepper.

3. Wrap each fillet as in a pouch, rolling foil down and sides up.

4. Place each pouch in a skillet and cook for 8–10 minutes on medium-low, or until the fish is opaque.

stuffed peppers

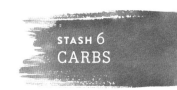

STASH 6
CARBS

1 cup short-grain brown rice

¼ cup wild rice

3 tablespoons plain Greek organic yogurt

3½ cups water

½ cup broth (chicken or beef)

1 teaspoon Real Salt

4 different-colored bell peppers

1 carrot

1 small onion

2 garlic cloves

1 tablespoon olive oil

1. The night before, place rice in a glass bowl. Add yogurt and 1½ cups of water. Mix and leave on the counter overnight. (This ferments the rice so it's easier to digest.)

2. The next day, rinse the rice in a strainer until the water runs clear Place the rice in a 4-quart saucepan. Add broth, 2 cups water, and salt. Cook on high until the rice begins to boil, then reduce flame to low, cover, and cook for 30 minutes, stirring occasionally Stir, then allow to cool.

3. Preheat over to 350°F. Cut off tops of peppers and core them. Wash out seeds. Mince carrot, onion, and garlic.

4. Heat olive oil in a sauté pan, then add carrot, onion, and garlic. Cook for 5 minutes, stirring occasionally. Add brown rice, then cook for another 2 minutes, stirring constantly.

5. Stuff rice mixture evenly into peppers. Place peppers on a baking sheet and roast for 20 minutes.

6. Allow to cool, then transfer to a glass container.

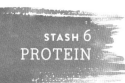

turkey meatballs

1 pound ground white-meat turkey
3 garlic cloves
2 tablespoons parsley
½ large yellow onion
2 teaspoons olive oil
½ cup Gluten-Free Almond Bread bread crumbs
Sea salt, to taste
Fresh-ground black pepper, to taste

1. Preheat oven to 350°F. Chop garlic and parsley. Mince the onion.

2. Heat olive oil in a pan, then add garlic and onions. Sauté until the onions are translucent.

3. Add ground turkey, breaking up the pieces with a large spoon and stirring constantly so it cooks evenly, about 7–10 minutes.

4. Remove from heat and place in a large bowl. Add bread crumbs and parsley. Mix with a large spoon (or your hands!) until the texture is even.

5. Shape into 8 2-ounce balls. Place on a baking sheet lightly greased with olive oil.

6. Place on the middle shelf in the oven. Bake for 10 minutes, turn each turkey ball over, then bake for 5–10 more minutes until the center is no longer pink.

7. Allow to cool, then transfer to a glass container.

8. Take two meatballs out and store in a separate container for meal 2 on Saturday. Cover the rest with Tomato Sauce.

TOMATO SAUCE

4 medium heirloom red tomatoes

6–8 cloves garlic

½ large yellow onion

2 tablespoons olive oil

½ cup (packed) fresh basil

1 teaspoon dried or ⅛ cup fresh oregano

1. Dice tomatoes. Chop the garlic and onion.

2. Heat olive oil in a large saucepan over medium heat. Sauté garlic and onions until onions are translucent.

3. Add basil and oregano. Sauté for about a minute, then add tomatoes.

4. Raise heat to medium-high and cook, stirring constantly, for 5–7 minutes.

5. Place mixture in a food processor or blender and blend until creamy.

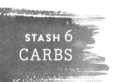

STASH 6
CARBS

quinoa noodles

3 cups quinoa noodles
1 teaspoon salt
1 teaspoon olive oil

1. Heat water to a boil with salt. Add noodles. Cook for 10 minutes. Noodles should be slightly al dente.

2. Transfer to a strainer and rinse with cold water to stop pasta from cooking. Shake off excess water and drizzle with a little olive oil to prevent sticking.

3. Allow to cool, then transfer to a glass container.

mashed cauliflower

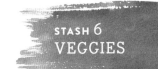

STASH 6
VEGGIES

2 medium heads cauliflower

1 cup water

½ cup broth (chicken or beef)

4 garlic cloves

¼ cup parsley, packed

1 teaspoon Real Salt

Fresh-cracked black pepper, to taste

1. Chop the cauliflower into small pieces. Place cauliflower in a stockpot with water, broth, and garlic. Bring to a boil and cook for 10 minutes.

2. Pour into a Vitamix blender or another type of powerful blender. Add parsley and salt. Blend, using the plunger, until smooth. Add pepper, to taste.

rainbow carrots

10 rainbow carrots

1 tablespoon flat-leaf Italian parsley

1 tablespoon olive oil

1 teaspoon sea salt

1 teaspoon fresh-ground black pepper

• • • • • • • •

Plain orange carrots are fine, too. We like rainbow for color.

1. Preheat oven to 350°F. Trim and quarter carrots. Chop the parsley. Mix all the ingredients on a baking sheet until the carrots are well coated with the oil. Use your hands!

2. Roast for 15 minutes, stir well, then roast for 10 more minutes.

3. Allow to cool, then transfer to glass containers.

STASH 6: MEAL PLAN

Thursday

MEAL 1

- 2 slices Gluten-Free Almond Bread
- ½ Hass avocado
- 2 eggs, prepared as you like them
  Make avocado toast, then top with eggs.

Snack

- 1 Granny Smith apple
- 2 tablespoon almond butter

MEAL 2

- 4 ounces Turkey Meatballs with Tomato Sauce
- 1 Stuffed Pepper
- 1 cup Mashed Cauliflower

Snack

- 1 cup blueberries
- 10 walnuts

MEAL 3

- 4 ounces Parcel-Poached Salmon
- ½ cup Quinoa Noodles with Tomato Sauce
- 1 cup Rainbow Carrots

Friday

MEAL 1

- 2 eggs, prepared as you like them
- 1 cup Mashed Cauliflower
- ½ cup Rainbow Carrots

Snack

- 1 cup blueberries
- 10 walnuts
- 1 tablespoon coconut flakes

MEAL 2

- 4 ounces Parcel-Poached Salmon
- ½ Hass avocado
- 1 Stuffed Pepper
- 2 cups butter lettuce
  Wrap salmon in lettuce top with avocado slices.

Snack

- 1 Granny Smith apple, sliced and sprinkled with cinnamon, if desired
- 10 walnuts

MEAL 3

- 4 ounces Turkey Meatballs
- 1 cup Rainbow Carrots
- ½ cup Quinoa Noodles with Tomato Sauce
- 2 cups spinach
- 1 tablespoon raw sunflower seeds

Saturday

MEAL 1

- 2 eggs, prepared as you like them
- 1 tablespoon real butter
- 1 cup Quinoa Noodles with Tomato Sauce

  Heat noodles and eggs together.

Snack

- 1 cup Mashed Cauliflower
- ½ Hass avocado
- 10 chopped almonds

MEAL 2

- wedding soup (see preparation, below)
- 1¼ cups broth
- 4 ounces Turkey Meatballs
- 1 cup spinach
- I carrot
- 1 slice toasted Gluten-Free Almond Bread
- ½ Hass avocado

  Heat broth with meatballs and spinach. Chop carrot and add.

Snack

- 1 Stuffed Pepper

MEAL 3

- 4 ounces Parcel-Poached Salmon
- 1 cup Mashed Cauliflower
- ½ cup Quinoa Noodles with Tomato Sauce
- 1 tablespoon olive oil
- 1 tablespoon raw sunflower seeds

  Top 2 cups of butter lettuce with salmon, noodles, and seeds.

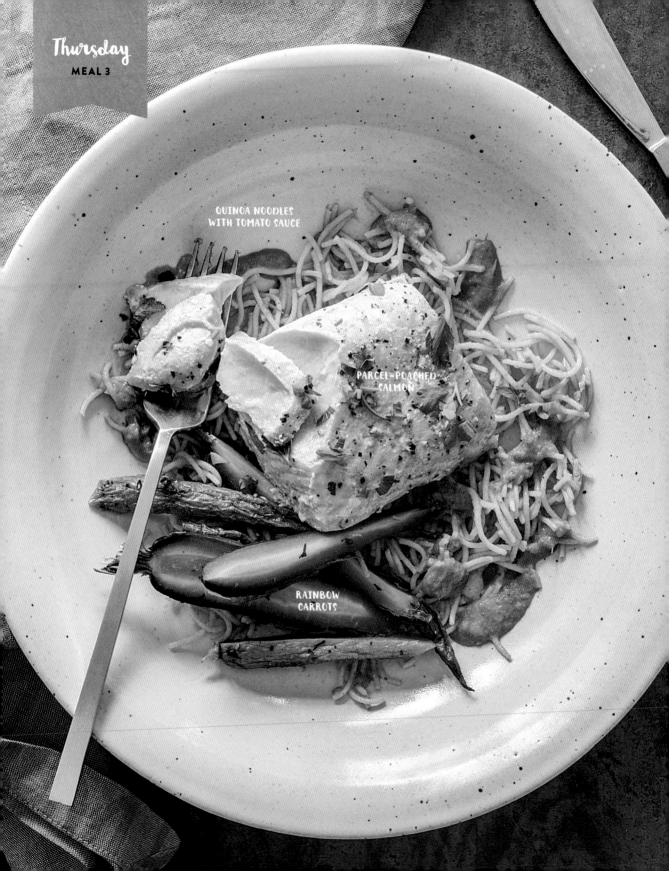

QUINOA NOODLES
WITH TOMATO SAUCE

PARCEL-POACHED
SALMON

RAINBOW
CARROTS

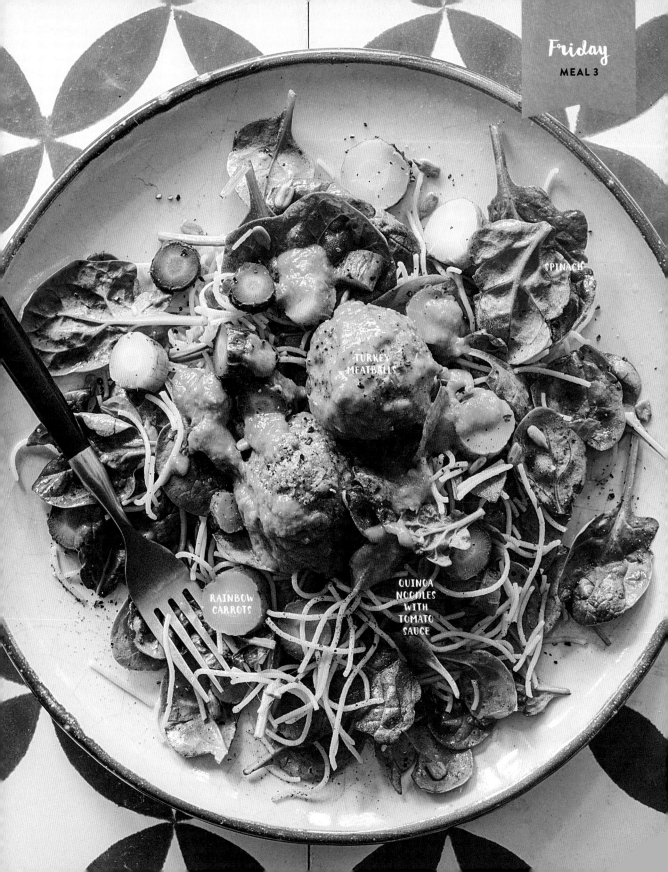

SPINACH

TURKEY
MEATBALLS

RAINBOW
CARROTS

QUINOA
NOODLES
WITH
TOMATO
SAUCE

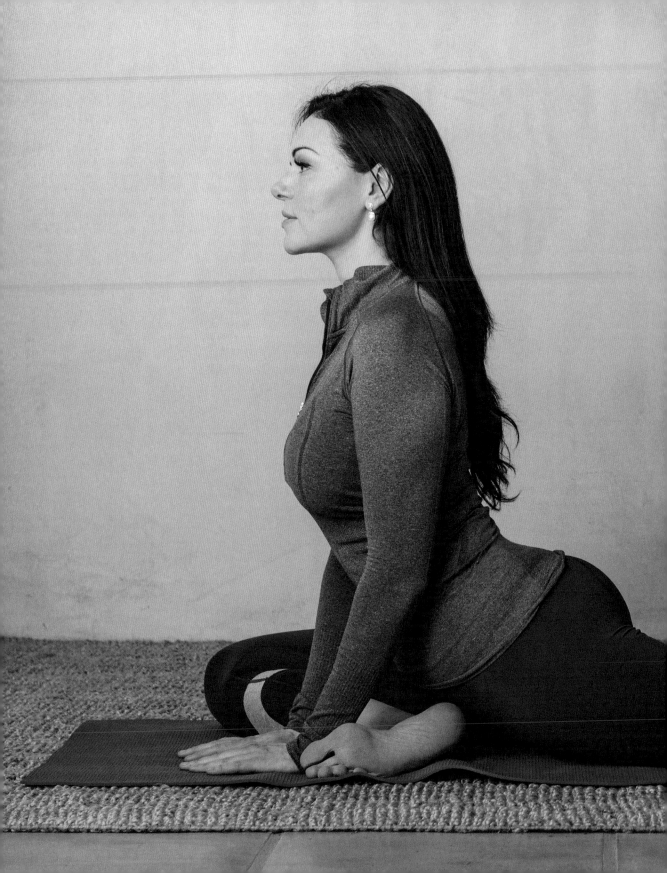

Stash Stretching

Targeted STRETCHING TO UNLOCK YOUR Natural-born ENERGY

chapter 12

ARE YOU READY TO FEEL BETTER?

With only a few minutes of *stretching* each day, you are going to have incredible results. These aren't typical stretches—they *unblock* your qi and *untangle* your fascia and improve your overall health and well-being. *So let's get to it.*

Stretch 1
Gallbladder Hurdler's Stretch

STEP 1: GETTING INTO POSITION

Lie down on your back on your mat. Bend both legs, placing your left foot on the ground and bringing your right leg toward your chest. Place your right arm on the outside of your right leg. Reach for your right ankle with your left hand.

STEP 2: RESISTANCE

Start with your leg and ankle out away from your body. Continuously push your right ankle and knee away from your body as you pull back with your right arm and your left arm, resisting against the ankle and knee.

STEP 3: REPETITION

Slowly bring your right leg down to the floor. Repeat Step 1 on your left side.

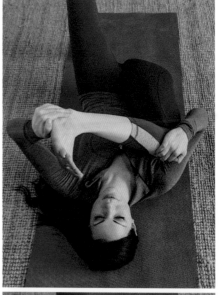

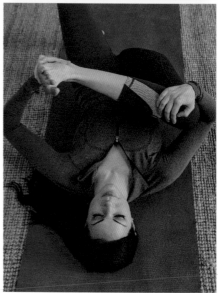

Stretch 2
Hamstring Lengthening Liver

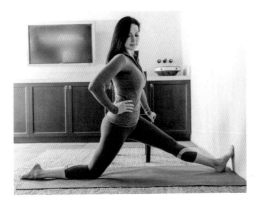

STEP 1: GETTING INTO POSITION

Place your mat against a wall. Stand on the end of it, facing the wall. Carefully come to a kneeling position. Extend your right leg so that your toes are touching the wall, making sure your foot is flexed and your heel is pressing down. Your left knee should be aligned with your left hip. If need be, you may add an extra mat under your knee to relieve pressure.

STEP 2: RESISTANCE

Pull back through the heel of your extended leg, while pushing forward with your kneeling leg, working in opposition.

STEP 3: REPETITION

Slowly revert to your original position, standing on the end of the mat. Repeat Steps 1 and 2 on your left leg.

Stretch 3
Spinal Extension

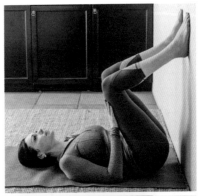

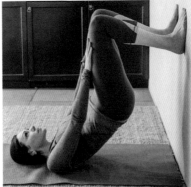

STEP 1: GETTING INTO POSITION

Sit on the end of your mat and scoot your glutes so they press against the wall. Next, lie down flat and bring your feet flat against the wall. Bring your hands to your knees and simultaneously lift your pelvis and back upward.

STEP 2: RESISTANCE

Your feet should not move position but should be pushing upward for resistance. Slowly roll down the wall one vertebrae at a time until your back is flat on the mat again.

STEP 3: REPETITION

Repeat 10 times.

Stretch 4
Gallbladder Hip Stretch

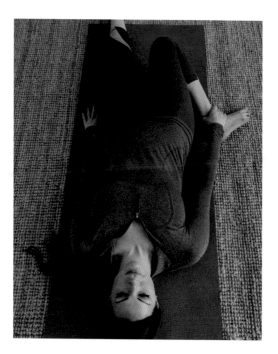

STEP 1: GETTING INTO POSITION
Lie down flat on your back on your mat. Your left leg remains straight on the mat while pressing down into the floor. Shift your right leg 45 degrees to the side. Next, bend your right leg, dragging your heel to your right hand. Grasp your right ankle in your right hand, holding your ankle as close to your upper thigh and glutes as possible.

STEP 2: RESISTANCE
Hold your right ankle stationary while drawing your right knee down toward the mat.

STEP 3: REPETITION
Continue creating resistance and pumping your leg back and forth. Repeat on your left side 8 times

Stretch 5
Squatting Liver

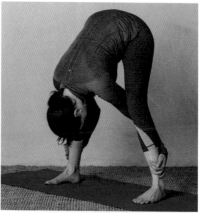

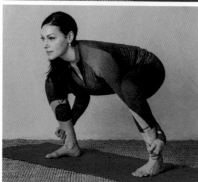

STEP 1: GETTING INTO POSITION
Stand with your feel parallel and slightly wider than shoulder width apart. Bend forward, reaching both hands between your legs and grabbing the outside of both ankles. Next, bend your knees, squatting down and lifting your head up and forward.

STEP 2: RESISTANCE
Pull up with your hands on your ankles, and press in with your knees against your arms and shoulders. Slowly straighten your legs, continuing to resist, keeping your head in line with your spine.

STEP 3: REPETITION
Repeat 10 times.

Stretch 6
Gallbladder Quad Stretch

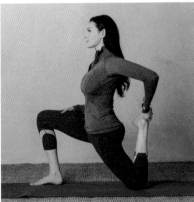

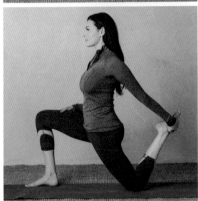

STEP 1: GETTING INTO POSITION
Kneel on your mat. Bend your right leg in front of you at a 90-degree angle. Keep your left knee bent under your hip. Put your right hand on your right knee. Reach back with your left hand and grasp the top of your left foot, keeping your torso upright.

STEP 2: RESISTANCE
Kick backward with your left foot while pulling with your left hand. Use your right hand pressing against your right leg for stability.

STEP 3: REPETITION
Repeat 5 times on each side.

Stretch 7
Kneeling Liver

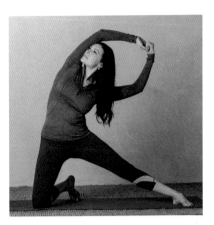

STEP 1: GETTING INTO POSITION
Kneel facing the long side of your mat. Extend your left leg directly to the side with toes pointing forward. Lift your arms above your head. Stack your hands palm to palm with your left hand over your right, and clasp hands together. Bend sideways over to the left, directly over the extended leg.

STEP 2: RESISTANCE
Pull down with your left arm and pull away with your right, working in opposition. While pulling with your arms, look up and open up your chest by rotating slightly to the right.

STEP 3: REPETITION
Repeat 5 times on each side.

Stretch 8
Gallbladder Psoas Stretch

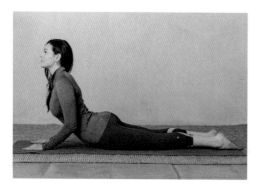

STEP 1: GETTING INTO POSITION

Lie down flat facing the top of your mat. Bring your palms directly under your shoulders, elbows pulling in toward your back. Squeeze your ankles together, pressing the tops of your feet into the floor.

STEP 2: RESISTANCE

Contracting your feet, legs, and glutes, push your hands into the floor, lifting your torso off the floor while pushing your pelvis into the mat. Continue pushing down with your hands while simultaneously pulling your arms back to create resistance. Slowly lower yourself down to original position.

STEP 3: REPETITION

Repeat 5 times.

Stretch 9
The Gallbladder Twist

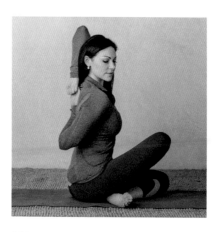

STEP 1: GETTING INTO POSITION

Sit cross-legged on your mat. Lift your left arm up and bend it so you can place your palm in the middle of your upper back. Reach your right arm back and bend it up to meet your right hand.

STEP 2: RESISTANCE

Pull up with your left hand and pull down with your right, creating tension.

STEP 3: REPETITION

Repeat 5 times on each side.

Stretch 10
Sitting Gallbladder

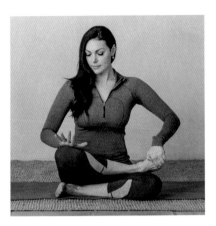

STEP 1: GETTING INTO POSITION
Sit on your mat. Bend your left leg in, and place your right leg on top on your left, right foot on top of your left knee. Keep both feet flexed.

STEP 2: RESISTANCE
Lift your right knee up as high as possible, then place your right palm on top of your right knee and press down, working in opposition.

STEP 3: REPETITION
Repeat 10 times on each side.

Stretch 11
Seated Liver

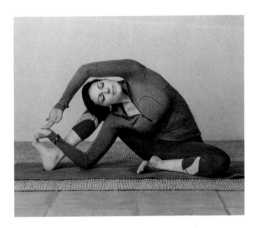

STEP 1: GETTING INTO POSITION
Sit sideways, close to the end of your mat. Extend your right leg to the right side, keeping your left leg bent in. Slightly bend your right knee and flex your right foot. Drop your right shoulder and extend your right arm inside your right leg, pressing your shoulder into your knee and keeping your palm facing upward. Place your left hand on your left knee. Grasp your big toe with your pointer and middle fingers.

STEP 2: RESISTANCE
Push down with your left hand, and push up with your left knee in opposition. Press your right knee and right shoulder against each other. To take it to the next level, reach your left arm over your head and grasp your right thumb while pulling back with your left hand. Rotate your torso out, bringing your head through the opening in your arms.

STEP 3: REPETITION
Repeat 5 times on each side.

Stretch 12
Folded Liver

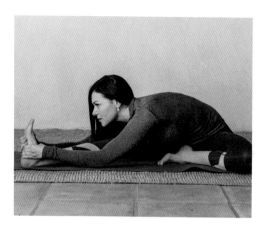

STEP 1: GETTING INTO POSITION

Sit facing the long end of your mat, close to the end. Extend your right leg to the right side, keeping your left leg bent in. Flex your right foot, extend your right arm down the outer side of your right leg, and extend your left arm down the inside of your right leg. Reach down as far as you can with both hands, and grasp onto your leg or foot.

STEP 2: RESISTANCE

Press your heel down into the floor and pull back toward your body with your hands still grasping your leg or foot. To take it a step further, bend your torso down and touch your forehead to your leg.

STEP 3: REPETITION

Repeat 5 times on both sides.

Stretch 13
Full Body Gallbladder into Liver Land

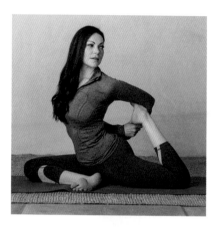

STEP 1: GETTING INTO POSITION

Sit at the top of your mat. Bend your right leg in and extend your left leg backward, shifting your weight forward. Extend your arms straight under your shoulders with your fingers pointing forward and your palms flat against the mat.

STEP 2: RESISTANCE

Press down and away with your right leg, then press your left leg into the floor from your foot all the way to your thigh. Push down and back with your palms, and arch your back up, looking toward the ceiling. To take it a step further, bend your left knee, and reach back with your left hand and grasp your left foot from the outside. Pull your left leg in with your left arm, simultaneously bending your elbow to create tension while pressing your left thigh into the floor.

STEP 3: REPETITION

Change to right leg in front and go through the stages 4 times on each side.

Stretch 14
Wall Gallbladder

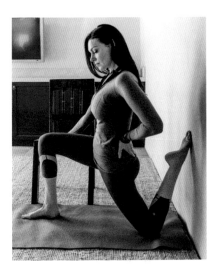

STEP 1: GETTING INTO POSITION
Place a chair on the right side of your mat for
balance. Kneel on your mat, facing away from the
wall. Slide your left knee back, toward the wall,
and rest the top of your left foot against the wall.
Extend your right leg forward and in front of you,
bending it at a right angle.

STEP 2: RESISTANCE
Push down and away with your right foot while
pulling forward with your left knee. If you are
having a hard time balancing you can use the chair
on your right for support.

STEP 3: REPETITION
Repeat 5 times on both sides.

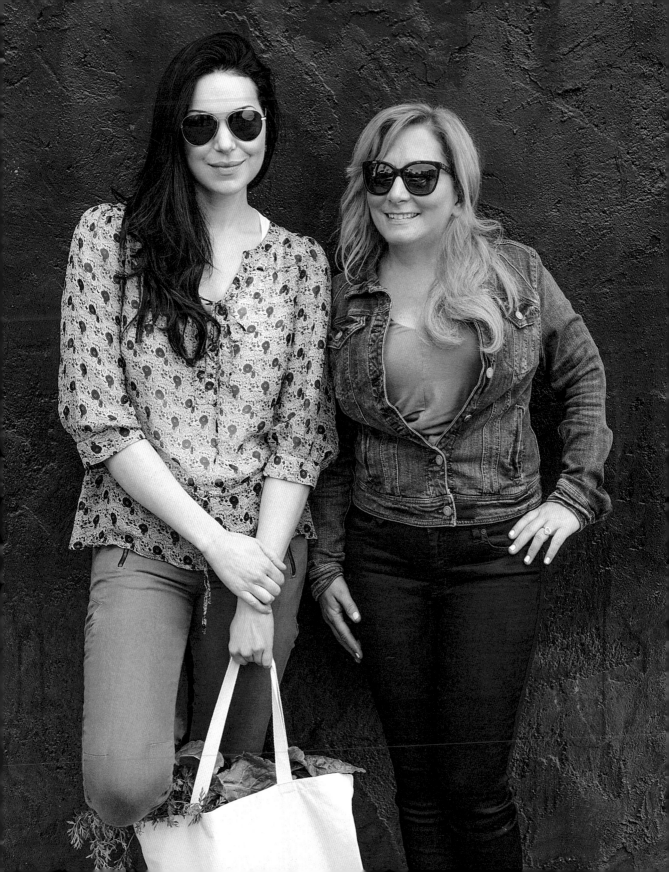

Conclusion

Now that you have made Stashing a part of your daily life, you are well on your way to becoming that lean mean sexy machine!

We've taught many people how to Stash, and they soon realize that the key to Stashing is its simplicity. Stashers get into the groove of preparing their Stashes, and once they do, they notice how much easier food shopping is, how stress is eliminated from their lives because there is no more worrying about what and where to eat. They start feeling better and looking better, their skin starts improving and their energy is higher. They say good-bye to prepared and packaged foods that were making them feel awful and sluggish and making their waistline expand.

You'll get so used to taking your Stashes to work or wherever you need to be that you won't remember wanting to eat any other way. You'll find yourself doing the stretches that work so well as soon as you get up in the morning. You'll be doing them at work when you're taking a break (and showing your coworkers what to do). You'll want to do them at night so you can unwind before bedtime. They're going to become just another part of your day, as vital to you as brushing your teeth and kissing your children good night.

And of course those pounds will be gone—and they'll stay gone.

Most of all, making your Stashes is *fun.* How you'll be eating will never feel like one of those umpteen diets you've tried before—diets that are all about deprivation and denial. Feel free to play around with your Stashes! Figure out what your personal go-tos are. Share recipes with friends and family. You don't have to give up anything you really love, because as long as you're Stashing on an 80/20 schedule, you'll be able to have those cocktails with your friends or a piece of cheesecake when the cravings really hit. And what you'll eventually see is that the cravings soon diminish altogether and your appetite stabilizes. Laura doesn't even need her hand grabbers anymore!

HAPPY STASHING!

Acknowledgments

LAURA

My family: Mommy, Stephanie, Jocelyn, Dani, Brad, James, Sebi, and Greg (and in loving memory of Daddy). Thank you for always supporting me in all my endeavors and for your unwavering belief in me. I love you. Mommy, you inspire me to always reach for the stars and to never conform to the status quo.

My second family: Jodi, Terasa, Camilla, and Rebecca . . . my best friends, my Silly Bs. Thank you for your support and awesomeness. You guys mean the world to me, and I know no matter what, we will always be there for each other. Love you.

Our team at Simon & Schuster and our editor, Michelle Howry, at Touchstone: Thank you so much for believing in us. This book will help so many people, and I so appreciate you seeing our vision and our message. Go, Team Stash!

Folio Literary Management: Frank and Dado! You guys are awesome. Thank you for taking us on. I know we broke the mold you are used to and I thank you for trusting us and coming with us on this journey!

Karen Moline: Thanks so much for all your contributions to the book and for being there with us on this awesome journey.

Elizabeth Troy, my coauthor: Thank you for entrusting me with your knowledge and believing in me in our collaboration. I love our book so much and am extremely proud of our work together. You rock, girl!

ELIZABETH

My daughter, Madeleine Troy:
Thank you for your patience for our
world to catch up and pay attention.
Lead the way and continue the positive
movement. I am so proud of the woman
you've become. I love you more than
the universe!

My man, Watts Wacker: Through
your love, support, and guidance you
have been the force to make all this
happen. I am so in love with you!

My mother, Marylyn Smith: Thank
you for your unconditional belief in me
and my work. At almost eighty years
old, having raised five children on your
own, you are an inspiration to all!

My coauthor, Laura Prepon:
Wow! Thank you for your trust and
perseverance throughout all our work
together. This book is a catalyst of
goodness. The combination of our
energy will help many!

**The team at Simon & Schuster
and our editor, Michelle Howry,
at Touchstone:** Your energy and
dedication to our passion has
made this a wonderful experience
come to life!

Karen Moline: Thank you
for your wonderful work and
guidance on *The Stash Plan*!

**Folio Literary Management and
our agents, Frank Weimann
and Dado Derviskadic:** The first
meeting said it all. The four of us
clicked. Our first book is just the
beginning. So much fun!

Index

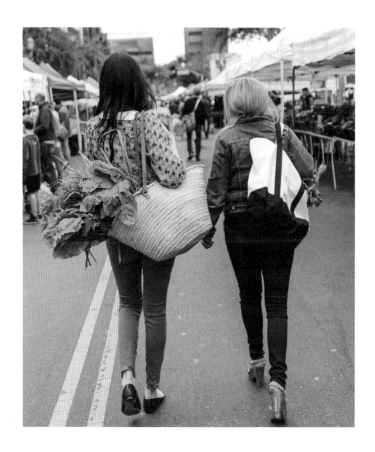

About the Authors

LAURA PREPON is a versatile actress whose career spans both film and television. She made her television debut on the long-running sitcom *That '70s Show*, and she can now be seen in the hit Netflix original series *Orange Is the New Black*. In addition to her acting work, Laura has had a lifelong passion for health and wellness, which has culminated in the creation of this book. An East Coaster at heart, Laura's home base is currently Los Angeles.

ELIZABETH TROY is the founder of Peak Experience NYC and the creator of Muscle Meridian Method, LLC. Her practice specializes in self-created healing. Elizabeth splits her time between Connecticut and New York City.